Fatal
Freedom

Books by Thomas Szasz

Pain and Pleasure
The Myth of Mental Illness
Law, Liberty, and Psychiatry
Psychiatric Justice
The Ethics of Psychoanalysis
The Manufacture of Madness
Ideology and Insanity
The Age of Madness (ed.)
The Second Sin
Ceremonial Chemistry
Heresies
Karl Kraus and the Soul Doctors
Schizophrenia
Psychiatric Slavery
The Theology of Medicine
The Myth of Psychotherapy
Sex by Prescription
The Therapeutic State
Insanity
The Untamed Tongue
Our Right to Drugs
A Lexicon of Lunacy
Cruel Compassion
The Meaning of Mind

Fatal Freedom

The Ethics and Politics of Suicide

THOMAS SZASZ

PRAEGER

Westport, Connecticut
London

Library of Congress Cataloging-in-Publication Data

Szasz, Thomas Stephen, 1920–
    Fatal freedom : the ethics and politics of suicide / Thomas Szasz.
      p. cm.
    Includes bibliographical references and index.
    ISBN 0–275–96646–1 (alk. paper)
    1. Suicide—Moral and ethical aspects. I. Title.
   HV6545.S89   1999
   179.7—dc21   99–13525

British Library Cataloguing in Publication Data is available.

Library of Congress Catalog Card Number: 99–13525
ISBN: 0–275–96646–1

First published in 1999

Praeger Publishers, 88 Post Road West, Westport, CT 06881
An imprint of Greenwood Publishing Group, Inc.
www.praeger.com

Printed in the United States of America

The paper used in this book complies with the
Permanent Paper Standard issued by the National
Information Standards Organization (Z39.48–1984).

10 9 8 7 6 5 4 3 2 1

Suicide is an event that is a part of human nature. However much may have been said and done about it in the past, every person must confront it for himself anew, and every age must come to its own terms with it.

Der Selbstmord ist ein Ereignis der menschlichen Natur, welches, mag auch darüber schon viel gesprochen und gehandelt sein als da will, doch einen jeden Menschen zur Teilnahme fordert, in jeder Zeitepoche wieder einmal verhandelt werden muss.

—Johann Wolfgang von Goethe (1749–1832),
Dichtung und Wahrheit (Poetry and Truth), p. 637; *The Truth and Fiction Relating to My Life*, in *The Complete Works of Johann Wolfgang von Goethe*, vol. 2, p. 163. Freely translated by Thomas Szasz. John Oxenford offers this translation: "Suicide is an event of human nature, which, whatever may be said and done with respect to it, demands the sympathy of every man, and in every epoch must be discussed anew."

Contents

Preface

[Cicero] has left it on record that he always studied his adversary's case with as great, if not still greater, intensity than even his own. What Cicero practiced as the means of forensic success requires to be imitated by all who study any subject in order to arrive at the truth. He who knows only his own side of the case, knows little of that.

—John Stuart Mill (1806–1873)[1]

Behind Goethe's simple statement lies a profound truth: Dying voluntarily is a *choice* intrinsic to human existence. It is our ultimate, fatal freedom. But that is not how the right-thinking person today sees voluntary death: He believes that no one in his right mind kills himself, that suicide is a mental health problem. Behind that belief lies a transparent evasion: relying on physicians to prevent suicide, prescribe suicide, and provide suicide—and thus avoid the subject of suicide. It is an evasion fatal to freedom.

Let us remember that not long ago the right-thinking person believed that masturbation, homosexuality, oral sex, and other "unnatural acts" were medical problems whose solutions were delegated to doctors. It took us a surprisingly long time to take these behaviors back from physicians—to accept them comfortably, to speak about them calmly, and to distinguish clearly between phenomena and judgments, descriptions and denunciations. One of my aims in this book is to help us accept suicide comfortably, to enable us to speak about it calmly, and to distinguish clearly between describing and condemning (or recommending) dying voluntarily. To accomplish this, we must demedicalize and destigmatize voluntary death and accept it as a behavior that has always been and will always be a part of the human condition. Wanting to die or killing oneself is sometimes blameworthy, sometimes praiseworthy, and sometimes neither; it is not a disease and it cannot be a *bona fide* medical treatment; and it is never adequate justification for coercion by the State.

Increasing life expectancy, advances in medical technology, and radical changes in the regulation of drug use and the economics of health care have transformed how we die. Formerly, most people died at home; now most people die in a hospital. Formerly, patients who could not breathe or whose kidneys, livers, or hearts failed to function died; now they can be kept alive by machines, transplanted organs, and immunosuppressive drugs. These developments have created choices not only about whether to live or die, but also about when and how to die. If we delegate responsibility for making these choices to medical professionals, we take a giant step toward forfeiting our basic freedoms.

Birth and death are unique phenomena. Celibacy or infertility notwithstanding, practicing birth control—that is, procreating voluntarily—is a personal decision. Accidental or sudden death notwithstanding, practicing death control—that is, dying voluntarily—should also be a personal decision.[2] The State and the medical profession no longer interfere with birth control. They ought to stop interfering with death control. Practicing birth control and practicing death control as well as abstaining from these practices have far-reaching consequences, both for the individual and for others. Birth control is important for the young; death control, for the old. The young are often entrapped by abstaining from birth control; the old, by abstaining from death control.

As individuals, we can choose to die actively or passively, practicing death control or dying of disease or old age. As a society, we can choose to let people die on their own terms or force them to die on terms decreed by the dominant ethic. Camus maintained that suicide is the only "truly serious philosophical problem."[3] It would be more accurate to say that suicide is our foremost moral and political problem, logically anterior to such closely related problems as the right to reject treatment or the right to physician-assisted suicide.

Faced with a particular personal conduct, we can approve, facilitate, and reward it; disapprove, hinder, and penalize it; or accept, tolerate, and ignore it. Over time, social attitudes toward many behaviors have changed: What was once regarded as a sin might become a crime or an illness or a life style or a constitutional right or even a treatment. Suicide began as a sin, became a crime, then became a mental illness, and now some people propose transferring it into the category called "treatment," provided the "cure" is under the control of doctors.

Is killing oneself a voluntary act or the product of mental illness? Should physicians be permitted to forcibly prevent suicide? Should they be authorized to prescribe a lethal dose of drug for the purpose of suicide? Should they practice mercy killing? Personal careers, professional identities, multibillion-dollar industries, legal doctrines, judicial procedures, and the life and liberty of every American hangs on how we answer these questions. Formulating an answer requires no specialized knowledge of Medicine or Law. It requires only a willingness to open our eyes and look life—and death—in the eye. Evading that challenge is tantamount to denying that we are just as responsible for how we die as we are for how we live.

The person who kills himself sees suicide as a *solution*. If the observer views it as a *problem*, he precludes understanding the suicide just as surely as he would preclude understanding a Japanese speaker if he assumed that he is hearing garbled English. For the person who kills himself or plans to kill himself, suicide is, *eo ipso*, an action. Psychiatrists, however, maintain that suicide is a happening, the result of a disease: As coronary arteriosclerosis causes myocardial infarction, so clinical depression causes suicide. Set against this mind-set, the view that suicide has nothing to do with illness or medicine, advanced in these pages, risks being dismissed as an act of intellectual know-nothingness, akin to asserting that cancer has nothing to do with illness or medicine.

The evidence that suicide is *not* a medical matter is all around us. We are proud that suicide is no longer a crime, yet it is plainly not legal; if it were, it would be illegal to use force to prevent suicide and it would be legal to help a person kill himself. Instead, coercive suicide prevention is considered a life-saving treatment and helping a person kill himself is (in most jurisdictions) a felony. Supporters and opponents of policies concerning troubling social issues—such as slavery, pornography, abortion—have always invoked a sacred authority or creed to justify the policies they favored: formerly, God, the Bible, the Church; now, the Constitution, Law, Medicine. It is an unpersuasive tactic: Too many deplorable social policies have been justified by appeals to Scriptural, Constitutional, and Medical sanctions.

One of the most troubling issues we face today is who should *control* when and how we die. The debate is in full swing, the participants again invoking the authority of the Bible, the Constitution, and Medicine to cast the decisive ballot in favor of their particular program. It is a spineless gambit: People who promote particular social policies do so because they believe that their policies are superior to the policies of their adversaries. Accordingly, they ought to defend their position on the grounds of their own moral vision instead of trying to disarm opponents by appealing to a sanctified authority.

For a long time, suicide was the concern of the Church and the priest. Now it is the business of the State and the doctor. Eventually we will make it our own choice, regardless of what the Bible or the Constitution or Medicine supposedly tells us.

Acknowledgments

I am deeply grateful to Peter Uva, librarian at the SUNY Health Science Center at Syracuse, for his generous help, year after year, book after book.

Alice Michtom gave me much useful advice and tireless help with revising and re-revising the manuscript.

Robert Schneebeli and Roger Yanow read the entire manuscript, sometimes in more than one version, and offered valuable suggestions.

Leo Elliott, Arthur Fliney, Charles Howard, David Levy, and Jeffrey Schaler helped with the initial drafts, sent clippings, and suggested references.

Nancy Cummings helped with the section on suicide by discontinuing hemodialysis.

My brother George, daughters Susan Palmer and Margot Peters, and son-in-law Steve Peters, each in his or her way, helped with the writing of the book by giving me their love and devotion.

I wish to express my heartfelt thanks to all of them and the many others not named who have supported my work in ways small and large.

Speaking of Suicide
Our Self-Mutilated Vocabulary

Whoever kills himself is a murderer, for the commandment "Thou shalt not kill" implies a general prohibition of killing human beings, "neither another, nor yourself."

—St. Augustine (354–430)[1]

Suicide: one who dies by his own hand; one who commits self-murder; the act or an act of taking one's own life, self-murder.

—*The Oxford English Dictionary* (1971)

Suicide: an act or an instance of taking one's own life voluntarily and intentionally.

—*Webster's Third New International Dictionary* (1971)

Everyone dies of something—old age, illness, injury, homicide, or suicide. Although most people are squeamish about dying, nearly everyone accepts death due to old age, disease, accident, and even murder as understandable or "normal." Suicide is a different matter: Killing oneself is generally viewed with abhorrence (sometimes with reverence) and the act of deliberately causing one's own death is treated as spooky, defying understanding, something "abnormal" or better not spoken or thought about. We are so phobic about suicide that we even fear reading about it. According to a 1992 poll, 71 percent of Americans want libraries to ban "books describing how to commit suicide."[2]

Having rejected self-killing as *a priori* wrong, we have mutilated our language: For killing others, we have a richly nuanced vocabulary; for killing ourselves, we have only a single word, which we hate to utter. We can ill afford this linguistic self-paralysis: Thinking clearly and speaking honestly about novel existential options posed by novel conditions of dying require expanding our vocabulary so that we can distinguish among different forms of voluntary deaths and their manifold meanings.

Is refusing food—as practiced by hunger strikers and persons diagnosed with anorexia nervosa—a form of suicide? Is withdrawal from hemodialysis and other life-sustaining treatments suicide? Does physician-assisted suicide count as suicide? Does a doctor killing a patient with the patient's consent—called "voluntary euthanasia"—count as suicide? Does a doctor killing a patient without the patient's consent but in his own best interest—called simply "euthanasia"—count as suicide? Is suicide legal? Should it be legal? If not, how should it be punished? If suicide is illegal but should not be punished, why should it be illegal? Is suicide a constitutional right? Should we treat it as if it were a right? We cannot grapple intelligently with these and similar questions so long as we systematically conflate and confuse phenomena and judgments, descriptions and evaluations.

Actually, we use the word "suicide" to express two quite different meanings: to *describe* a mode of death, that is, taking one's own life, voluntarily and deliberately; and to *denounce* the act, that is, to condemn it as sinful, criminal, irrational, unjustified, in a word, bad. Uncertain about the core meaning of the word "suicide," we cannot speak or think clearly about ending our own life.

Killing oneself or another person may be morally right or wrong or neither, depending on the circumstances and the values of the person doing the judging. In order to speak and think clearly about suicide, we must agree on its core meaning. I use the word "suicide" to refer to taking one's own life voluntarily and deliberately, either by killing oneself directly or by abstaining from a directly life-saving act; in other words, I regard any behavior motivated by a preference for death over life that leads directly (perhaps only after the lapse of several days) to the cessation of one's life as suicide. Whether we judge that act to be good or bad, rational or irrational, permissible or prohibited is important; but it is another matter.

LANGUAGE AND SUICIDE

We perceive and grasp reality through the mirror of language—the physical world, through the mirror of mathematical language, the human world, through the mirror of ordinary language. We know what we think by listening to our own (inner) voice. We infer what others think by listening to their voices. Let us begin by briefly examining the vocabularies in which people spoke about suicide in the past and speak about it now.

From Self-Killing to Suicide

In the ancient world people killed themselves by hanging, drowning, abstaining from food, jumping from a precipice, falling on their swords, supposedly even suffocating by holding their breath (if such accounts are to be believed).[3] In that faraway world, people regarded it as self-evident that taking a person's life—one's own or that of another—is a deliberate, voluntary act. Accordingly, the Greeks and Romans had only verbs and verbal nouns to describe what we call "suicide."[4] David Daube cogently notes that the term "suicide" came about as a way to avoid the accusing references to "murder."[5] The conceptual and linguistic transformation of "self-murder" into "dying by one's own hand" was the result of "an enhanced sophistication of mind and an improved technique for doing away with oneself [that is, the use of hemlock]."[6]

The ancient Greek language lacked a general expression for voluntary death but was rich in terms that name specific acts of self-killing. The comprehensive term for the deed was *autocheir*, "to act with one's own hand," an image that implies choice, planning, and self-determination, precisely the features that the modern bracketing of suicide with mental illness seeks to erase. Other terms for self-killing used various verbs, such as to "seize death," "grasp death," "break up life," "end life." Latin usage generally leaned on Greek precedent. The word *mors*, standing alone, meant dying involuntarily—as a result of accident, injury, disease, or old age. *Mors voluntaria*, the earliest noun phrase for voluntary death, is believed to be the creation of the Roman orator and statesman Marcus Tullius Cicero (106–43 B.C.).

When Shakespeare wrote, the word "suicide" was not yet a part of the English language. Robert Burton, the author of *Anatomy of Melancholy* (1652), does not use the word "suicide"; nor does John Milton in *Paradise Lost* (1667) or in *Samson Agonistes* (1671).[7] According to *The Oxford English Dictionary*, the term was first used in 1651; that entry reads: "To vindicate ones self from . . . inevitable Calamity, by Suicide is . . . not a crime"; an even more remarkable entry, dated 1730, states: "The Suicide owns himself. . . ." Until the middle of the seventeenth century, "good writers use *self-homicide*, never *suicide*."[8] In the nineteenth century, writers begin to legitimize some types of voluntary death by replacing the word "suicide" with phrases like "death by choice," "self-deliverance," "mercy death," and "euthanasia."

The appearance of the *noun* "suicide," like the term "mind" as a noun, is a seventeenth-century Western invention.[9] Both terms reflect a major cultural-perceptual shift: from perceiving voluntary death as an act for which the actor is responsible, to perceiving it as a (perhaps) happening for which he may not be responsible; and from seeing persons as possessing souls and free will, to seeing them as possessing minds that may become "unbalanced," resulting in the loss of free will.

As long as self-killing was viewed as an act, language had only verbs and verbal nouns with which to name it. Absent the word "suicide," people viewed the self-killer as a moral agent, responsible for his deed. By contrast, we now think of suicide as a happening or result, attribute it to mental illness, and view the agent as a victim ("patient").

The transformation of soul into mind and self-murder into suicide marks the beginning of the great ideological transformation from religion to medicine—sins become sicknesses; "bad" behaviors that have motives (reasons) mutate into "mad" behaviors that have causes (etiologies). While attributing suicide to mental illness excuses and seemingly destigmatizes the act as the unintended consequence of illness, it incriminates and restigmatizes it as the manifestation of dreaded (hereditary) insanity.

The perception and interpretation of voluntary death as an unintended happening, similar to an unwanted illness, has two important consequences. One is that the person who tries but fails to kill himself is routinely diagnosed as depressed and deprived of liberty by being incarcerated in a mental hospital. The other is that the person who succeeds in killing himself while in a (mental) hospital or under the care of a mental health professional is considered to have died a "wrongful death," a victim for whose demise tort law holds his caretakers responsible.

The evolution of German and French words for suicide follows the familiar pattern, from rough verb to mild verb to abstract noun. The German noun *Selbstmord,* from the earlier *sich ermorden* ("to murder oneself"), first appeared in the seventeenth century. However, modern German is unique among Western languages in having a noun for noble suicide, *Freitod,* a shortened version of *freiwilliger Tod,* which translates literally as "freely willed death." That term effectively destigmatizes the act and shows willingness to consider some instances of voluntary deaths as rational and praiseworthy.

Like other words ending with the suffix "cide"—such as matricide, patricide, fratricide—the word "suicide" implies a wrongful act. Were we to call abortion "feticide" or "homicide in utero," we could not speak so casually about a woman's right to abortion. So long as we have only disapprobative terms for an act—such as "self-murder," "self-abuse," and "drug abuse"—we cannot grasp, and hence cannot study, the subjects they ostensibly describe, but actually de-mean. I use the word "de-mean" here to denote emptying the act or phenomenon of its rich meaning and imposing on it a single signification, typically of badness or madness. However, the other sense of de-meaning—that is, robbing the act (actor) of dignity and worth—applies as well. Although conventional wisdom regards medicalizing a (supposedly) problematic behavior and the interventions used to regulate it as evidence of ethical and scientific progress, it is nothing of the sort.

Two Types of Killing Persons: Heterohomicide and Autohomicide

We call the act of causing the death of a human being—by omission or commission—"homicide." Obviously, killing oneself differs radically from killing another person. Hence, the traditional, religion-inspired bracketing of self-murder with murder is misleading. To understand suicide, we must draw a clear distinction between killing oneself ("autohomicide") and killing another person ("heterohomicide").

Although we condemn homicide in the abstract, most people approve of certain types of killings, for example, self-defense or self-sacrifice. Moreover, all religions and cultures classify certain kinds of heterohomicide and autohomicide as laudable and praise them as "heroism" and "martyrdom." During World War II, the Japanese called their patriotic pilots "*Kamikaze*," which means Divine Wind;[10] we called them "suicide bombers." We translate the Other's experience and language into our own experience and language and delude ourselves that our misinterpretation *explains* the Other's behavior.[11]

We recognize that not every instance of heterohomicide is murder and we have a rich vocabulary to distinguish different types of killings, and vice versa. We call killing "murder" only if the actor's aim is to extinguish the other's life and his act is not otherwise legally justifiable. This enables us to distinguish murder from involuntary homicide, negligent homicide, and killing in self-defense. However, we generally use only one word for killing oneself, namely "suicide." This paucity of our vocabulary and our tendency to routinely attribute suicide to mental illness reflect our aversion to critical thinking about the subject. Although we recognize that the voluntary death of a young Japanese *Kamikaze* pilot is not the same sort of act as the suicide of an elderly American cancer patient, we resist understanding each act on its own terms: We prefer to explain away the act rather than grasp it by putting ourselves in the actor's place. Did the person who killed himself *want to die*? Was death the *end* he sought or only a *means* he chose to avoid dishonor, dependency, shame, suffering, and so forth? We refrain from asking such questions because we are afraid to confront suicide without the familiar religious and psychiatric defenses against it; because we are afraid to recognize that killing oneself is an existential option, perhaps even a moral obligation to ourselves and to others.

Judging Suicide

Suicide is morally problematic, and *ought to be* problematic, because it entails the *deliberate* killing of a human being. Hence, it needs to be judged. One option is to condemn it out of hand. Another is to treat it as we treat other types of killings, namely, by examining the context in which the act occurs, the actor's motives, and the consequences of his act.

Probably reflecting the fact that living is instinctively precious, no religion acknowledges the absolute finality of human life. We could, if we wanted to, attribute a nonsuicidal motive to every case of suicide, such as wanting to avoid physical pain or a painful life situation. However, asserting that no one wants to die, that persons who kill themselves do so only to avoid suffering, or that every suicide is an "unnecessary tragedy" that could be prevented—all these are facile and foolish denials of the inexorable reality and existential legitimacy of suicide.

In principle, killing oneself is not different from other acts that have far-reaching, irreversible consequences, such as begetting a child. The person who kills himself does so because he deems terminating his life preferable to continuing it. If we agree with his judgment, we call his suicide "rational"; if we do not, we call it "irrational."

The instinctive justification for killing another person (or beast) is self-defense. Reconciling the act with the seemingly unconditional prohibition of the commandment against "killing" presents a cognitive challenge whose resolution requires justifying self-defense itself.[12]* This is accomplished, most famously, by the so-called Principle of Double Effect. Because St. Thomas Aquinas (1225–1274) articulated this principle so eloquently in his *Summa Theologica*, he is usually credited with its origination. In a chapter titled "Whether it is lawful to kill a man in self-defense?" Aquinas justified the otherwise illicit act of killing as follows:

Nothing hinders one act from having two effects, only one of which is intended, while the other is beside the intention. Now moral acts take their species according to what is intended, and not according to what is beside the intention. Accordingly, the act of self-defense may have two effects, one is the saving of one's life, the other is the slaying of the aggressor. Therefore this act, since one's intention is to save one's own life, is not unlawful.[13]

By changing a few words, this formula may also be used to justify killing oneself, that is, suicide:

*Raising and resolving this dilemma appears to be closely connected with mankind's advance from a nonliterate to a literate mental state, creating, through the *written word*, a distinction between thought and action.

Nothing hinders one act from having two effects, only one of which is intended, while the other is beside the intention. Now moral acts take their species according to what is intended, and not according to what is beside the intention. Accordingly, the act of self-protection from depression, disability, and disease may have two effects, one is the protecting of one's bodily and mental integrity, the other is the killing of oneself. Therefore this act, since one's intention is to save one's own bodily and mental integrity, is not unlawful.[14]

The *New Catholic Encyclopedia* defines the Principle of Double Effect as follows: "A rule of conduct frequently used in moral theology to determine when a person may lawfully perform an action from which two effects follow, one bad, the other good."[15] For example, it is permissible for a Catholic woman to take birth control pills, provided her aim is not to prevent pregnancy but to regulate her menstrual cycle and relieve pain. Of course, there is nothing peculiarly Catholic about this mode of reasoning.

Paul Ramsey, an influential American Protestant writer on medical ethics, uses this argument to justify abortion. He writes: "Everything is lawful, *absolutely everything* is permitted which love permits, everything without a single exception. And *absolutely everything* is commanded which love requires, absolutely everything without the slightest exception or 'softening.' " Ramsey calls abortion "the *incapacitation* of the fetus from doing what it is doing to the life of the mother," and declares: "This distinction between incapacitation and direct killing solves the problem of explaining how love can justify abortion. If justifiable abortions are properly described as incapacitating rather than killing, then one can say that such actions are justifiable actions of love to the aborted fetus. One has not done something unloving to the fetus itself."[16]

Obviously, this sort of moral reasoning is infinitely elastic: It can be easily stretched to justify the self-serving act of any individual or group. For example, at the 1986 annual meeting of Sinn Fein,* a motion was passed "supporting the 'right to life,' with the exception that it should not apply to what they term the 'armed struggle.' "[17]

Because we human beings are language users through and through, everything we do is, *inter alia*, a message. The suicide sends a message, whether intended or not. Its recipient interprets it, whether he acknowledges doing so or not. Indeed, the fact that we insist on interpreting suicide as a message is the ultimate proof that we recognize it to be a deed, not a disease. If a young person dies of a ruptured aneurysm, we do not say that he *has done so to* make his family feel guilty; but if he dies of suicide, we sometimes make that accusation. The result is a virtually limitless variety of interpretations

Sinn Fein is Gaelic for "we ourselves" or "ourselves alone." It is the name of an Irish Nationalist society founded in 1905 and of the Irish Nationalist movement and party today.

of suicide, as blackmail, martyrdom, mental illness, medical treatment, self-liberation, and so forth.

Human behaviors—personal, sexual, social—are not medical matters. Killing oneself or others is behavior: It is a matter of ethics and politics. Attributing suicide to mental illness is merely the latest attempt to control and condemn voluntary death by medicalizing it.

Constructing Suicide
What Counts as Killing Oneself?

*That suicide may often be consistent with interest and with our duty to our-
selves, no one can question . . . I believe that no man ever threw away life, while
it was worth keeping.*
—David Hume (1711–1776)[1]

*Suicide being an act consecutive to the delirium of the passions or insanity . . .
[its] treatment belongs to the therapeutics of mental diseases.*
—Jean Etienne Dominique Esquirol (1772–1840)[2]

*[S]uicide, which amounts in rabbinic thought to murder, is strictly forbidden.
. . . However, recent rabbinic ruling considers the suicide as being of unsound
mind, and as such he is allowed to be interned [sic] with others.*
—The Encyclopedia of the Jewish Religion (1965)[3]

For almost two thousand years, the specter of suicide has haunted the Western mind. We have tried to exorcize that specter by the linguistic equivalent
of the ostrich's burying its head in the sand: By making ourselves unable to
speak clearly about voluntary death, we hope to unravel its mystery and
dispel its terror without having to look suicide in the face. As a result, there
is no general agreement about what counts as suicide, and when we speak
about it we say what we do not mean, and mean what we do not say.

We say that depression, guns, and tobacco kill people, but we mean that
persons we call "depressed" ought to see psychiatrists, that guns ought to
be outlawed, and that people ought not to smoke. We say that Smith is ill,
suffers, and has a right to physician-assisted suicide (PAS), but we mean
that people in Smith's position are better off dead, ought to be relieved of
the responsibility to kill themselves, and physicians ought to be authorized

to help them end their lives. The result is that we deceive ourselves and others to believe that depriving individuals of the opportunity to kill themselves, relieving them of responsibility to do so (if that is what they want), and giving physicians special powers to obstruct as well as to expedite suicide—while withholding such powers from everyone else—augment "patient autonomy."

HISTORY'S LESSONS

As we have seen, the Greeks and Romans could not conceive of dying voluntarily as unintentional, just as we cannot conceive of, say, skiing as unintentional. A popular Greek metaphor for the self-killer was the shipwrecked sailor who "swims away from the body and hopes to land in the safe haven of death."[4]

Because self-killing is an act with serious consequences not only for oneself, but for others as well, the Greeks and Romans judged it to be courageous or cowardly, noble or ignoble, legitimate or illegitimate, depending on the circumstances. Socrates believed that man was the property of the gods: Without their permission, self-killing was wrongful; with it, it was permissible, perhaps even praiseworthy. Plato (428–348 B.C.) interpreted the "visible necessity of dying" imposed on Socrates by the Athenian court as an instance of such divine permission, ennobling his voluntary death.

Because Plato's view of suicide prefigures the Christian view of it, it is worth citing his relevant comments.* In the *Phaedo*, Plato presents an account (attributed to Socrates's pupil Phaedo) of the philosopher's last hours, spent in conversation with friends. Reflecting on the predicament of a person who knows he has only a short time to live, Socrates observes that such a person, "like anyone else who is properly grounded in philosophy," would be willing to leave life voluntarily. "However," he adds, "he will hardly do himself violence, because they say it is not legitimate." This prompts his pupil Cebes to ask: "Socrates, what do you mean by saying that it is not legitimate to do oneself violence?"[5] Socrates replies:

The allegory which the mystics tell us—that we men are put in a sort of guard post, from which one must not release oneself or run away—seems to me to be a high doctrine with difficult implications. All the same, Cebes, I believe that this much is true, that the gods are our keepers, and we men are one of their possessions. . . . So if you look at it this way I suppose it is not unreasonable to say that we must not put an end to ourselves until God sends some compulsion like the one which we are facing now.[6]

*All we know about Socrates is what Plato tells us. His writings imply that he shared the ideas he attributes to Socrates.

The equanimity Socrates displays in the face of death is attributable partly to his firm belief in an afterlife superior to life on earth: "The man who has devoted his life to philosophy should be cheerful in the face of death [because he is] confident of finding the greatest blessing in the next world. . . . Since the soul is clearly immortal . . . it demands our care not only for that part of time which we call life, but for all time."[7] Edith Hamilton and Huntington Cairns, the editors of Plato's *Dialogues*, emphasize that "To himself Socrates was recovering, not dying. He was entering not into death, but into life, 'life more abundantly.' "[8]

Since the self-killer does wrong, what should be his punishment? In the *Laws* Plato answers: "The graves of such as perish thus must, in the first place, be solitary; they must have no companions whatsoever in the tomb. Further, they must be buried ignominiously in waste and nameless spots on the boundaries between the twelve districts, and the tomb shall be marked by neither headstone nor name."[9]

Aristotle (384–322 B.C.) reinforced the Platonic prohibition against suicide, asserting that man belongs not to himself but to the gods and the State. In the *Nicomachean Ethics*, he writes:

The law does not expressly permit suicide, and what it does not expressly permit it forbids. . . . [H]e who through anger voluntarily stabs himself does this contrary to the right rule of life, and this the law does not allow; therefore he is acting unjustly. But towards whom? Surely towards the state, not towards himself. For he suffers voluntarily, but no one is voluntarily treated unjustly. This is also the reason why the state punishes; a certain loss of civil rights attaches to the man who destroys himself, on the ground that he is treating the state unjustly.[10]

Roman law expanded the criteria that made suicide morally acceptable. For example, *taedium vitae*—a mental state we are likely to call "depression," but is better rendered as "having had enough (of life)"—was a justification for it.[11] However, Roman law prohibited the suicide of slaves, because they destroyed not themselves but their masters' property; and of defendants accused of crime, because their deed prevented the law from determining whether they were guilty or not. If their deed was *interpreted* as signifying guilt, the law required that their corpse be denied ritual burial and their property be confiscated. Christian canon law adopted the practice of denying religious burial to the suicide's corpse, and medieval English criminal law reinstated the penalty of forfeiting the suicide's property.[12]

Seneca (4 B.C.–A.D. 65), the most famous Stoic philosopher, rejected the paternalist-statist argument against suicide. He articulated what we now regard as the individualist-libertarian position on voluntary death, based on the right to self-ownership. "In whatever direction you may turn your eyes," he wrote, "there lies the means to end your woes. See you that precipice? . . . See you that sea, that well? There sits liberty—at the bottom." Seneca recommended suicide "when old age threatened to bring undignifying decay"[13] and warned that "maybe this should be done somewhat earlier than strictly is necessary to prevent you from being unable to do it when it has to be done."[14]

The Scripture writers recount several instances of justifiable self-killing. Saul, the first king of Israel, kills himself after the Philistines defeat his army, kill his sons, and wound him: "Therefore Saul took a sword, and fell upon it."[15] In the case of Samson's suicide, also occasioned by defeat, the motive is revenge. Delilah betrays him and the Philistines capture and blind him: whereupon "Samson said, Let me die with the Philistines. And he bowed himself with all his might; and the house fell upon the lords, and upon all the people that were therein."[16] In short, in biblical Jewish thought, as in Greco-Roman thought, self-killing in the interest of divine will is morally justified. Judas's suicide belongs in that class: "Then Judas, which had betrayed him . . . [said] to the chief priests and elders . . . I have sinned in that I have betrayed the innocent blood. And they said, What is that to us? See thou to that. And he cast down the pieces of silver in the temple, and . . . went and hanged himself."[17] Although Judas repents and seeks the forgiveness of the priests and elders, they do not chastise or punish him. They rebuff him. Judas must be his own judge and executioner.

After the Christianization of Rome, the Church adopted the Platonic principle that all human life belongs to God. The view that God gives and owns man's life and He, alone, has rightful authority to take it away lies at the heart of both the Jewish and Christian prohibitions against suicide as well as against contraception, abortion, and euthanasia. At the beginning of Christianity, this vision lead to the idea that dying for God is a way to demonstrate our love for Him. Saint Ignatius (d. c. A.D. 119), Bishop of Antioch, addressed these words to the Christian community of Rome: "I beseech you, suffer me to be eaten by the beasts . . . entice the wild beasts that they may become my tomb, and leave no trace of my body, that when I fall asleep I may be not burdensome to any. Then shall I be truly a disciple of Jesus Christ."[18] Gibbon viewed the deaths of early Christians who provoked the Roman authorities to kill them as suicides: "They [the early Christians] . . . cheerfully leaped into the fires . . . until the bishops themselves had to condemn such practices. 'Unhappy men!' exclaimed the proconsul of Asia, 'If you are thus weary of your lives, is it so difficult to find ropes and precipices?'"[19]

In A.D. 563, the Council of Braga declared suicide to be self-murder, punished by denial of burial in consecrated ground. In the Middle Ages, Christian sovereigns included the secular penalty of forfeiting the suicide's goods and property. A seventeenth-century observer offered this account of the burial of a suicide: "[The dead man] is drawn by a horse to the place of punishment and shame, where he is hanged on a gibbet, and none may take the body down but by the authority of the magistrate."[20] As recently as 1823, "a London suicide was buried at a cross-roads in Chelsea with a stake through his body."[21] The law of forfeiture remained in force in England until the nineteenth century, although, from the eighteenth century on, it was systematically circumvented by excusing the self-killer as *non compos mentis*.

Ecclesiastic law still forbids suicide, and religious penalties against the act are, nominally, still in force. However, as soon as secular law recognized insanity as an excuse for suicide, so, too, did canon law. For approximately the past century, rabbinic and church authorities alike have classified suicides as *ipso facto non compos*, permitting them to receive normal religious burial services. *The Encyclopedia of the Jewish Religion* states: "Judaism does not consider the individual as the owner or unlimited master of his own life; consequently, suicide, which amounts in rabbinic thought to murder, is strictly forbidden. . . . However, recent rabbinic ruling considers the suicide as being of unsound mind, and as such he is allowed to be interned [*sic*] with others."[22] The Roman Catholic Church and the Protestant clergy use the same formula for annulling the sinfulness of suicide. After a well-known Catholic American killed himself and was given an elaborate burial, a spokesman explained: "Today it is the church's feeling that a person must be crazy to commit suicide. And we place the insane in the hands of God, for his mercy and his judgment. . . . The church will not judge [him]."[23] Protestants use the same evasion, exonerating the suicide by defining him as a victim who committed the fatal deed "while the balance of his mind was disturbed."[24]

The Reformation exercised a complex and contradictory influence on the perception and interpretation of suicide. By restoring the authority of the Scriptures, Protestantism reinforced the belief that self-murder "was a terrible sin, caused directly by the Devil."[25] At the same time, by reembracing the Greco-Roman roots of Western civilization, the Reformation set the stage for the rediscovery of the idea that the individual is sovereign over himself, justifying suicide.

According to the Dutch humanist-scholar Desiderius Erasmus (c. 1466–1536), suicide was a legitimate escape from a troublesome world. He considered old people who killed themselves "wiser than those who are unwilling to die and want to live longer."[26] Michel de Montaigne (1533–1592) concluded: "After all, this life is ours, it is all we have."[27] Montesquieu (1680–1755) declared: "Life has been given to me as a gift . . . I can therefore return it when this is no longer the case. . . . When I am overwhelmed by pain, poverty and scorn, why does one want to prevent me from putting an end to my troubles, and to deprive me cruelly of a remedy which is in my hands?"[28]

John Donne (1573–1631), the poet dean of St. Paul's, in his posthumously published treatise, *Biathanatos* (1646), wrote: "Methinks I have the keys of my prison in mine own hand, and no remedy presents itself so soone to my heart, as mine own sword."[29] The Scottish philosopher David Hume (1711–1776) articulated the modern, secular-libertarian argument against religious and legal interference with suicide. In his *Essay on Suicide* (1783), also published posthumously, he argued that man owns himself and hence has a right to end his life: "Were the disposal of human life so much reserved as the peculiar province of the Almighty, that it were an encroachment on his right, for men to dispose of their own lives; it would be equally criminal to act for the preservation of life as for its destruction. . . . If my life be not my own, it were criminal for me to put it in danger, as well as to dispose of it."[30] Voltaire (1694–1778), Goethe (1749–1832), and Schopenhauer (1788–1860) held similar views.[31]

However, there was certainly no shortage of defenders of the prohibition against suicide, the most prominent among them being Immanuel Kant (1724–1804). He declared: "If freedom is the condition of life, it cannot be employed to abolish life and so to destroy and abolish itself . . . suicide is in no circumstances permissible. . . . Moral philosophers must, therefore, first and foremost show that suicide is abominable."[32] *Mutatis mutandis*, psychiatrists believe that it is their first and foremost duty to show that suicide is abnormal.

MEDICALIZING SUICIDE

With the exception of *public health*, the history of medicine (until recently) has been the history of *private health*, a phrase I use here to underscore the distinction between two radically different kinds of *medical situations and services*. The term "public health" refers to measures intended to benefit the health of the general population (or a large group), not that of any particular individual regarded as a patient (for example, providing a safe system of sewage disposal); whereas the term "private health" refers to a *consensual relationship* between doctor and patient, the former providing medical care to the latter (for example, removing a person's inflamed appendix).

The systematic isolation of individuals formally identified as insane constitutes a radical departure from the principle that, in the absence of the patient's consent, medical intervention is a form of assault and battery. This practice was justified as the *prevention of harm by the self to self*, adding, for good measure, that the practice also serves to prevent the insane person from harming others (and is therefore justifiable on the model of quarantining individuals with contagious diseases). In this way, the *use of physicians by the State* as well as the *use of force by physicians* was extended from public health to mental health, initially called "mad-doctoring," now called "psychiatry." By the end of the eighteenth century, when King George III was managed by mad-doctors, forcible detention and restraint were accepted methods for treating the insane.[33]

Initially, mad persons were detained in a space not called a "hospital" and their detention was called "confinement"; the restraint was mechanical and was called the "strait-waistcoat" in England, and the "straitjacket" in America. In England the mad-doctors' patients/prisoners were upper-class persons unwanted by their relatives, while in France they were lower-class persons unwanted by society. Now, detention is in a medical facility and is called "hospitalization"; the restraint is chemical and is called "medication" or "drug treatment"; and potentially everyone—regardless of age or class or gender—is eligible to be the psychiatrists' patient/prisoner. Once again, being a "suicidal risk" is rapidly becoming the only generally accepted justification for inpatient psychiatric treatment," that is, for psychiatric detention.[34]

During the French Revolution, the State forged a close alliance with medicine and replaced legal controls of behavior with coercions defined as "medical procedures." Animated by anticlerical zeal, the Jacobins repealed the law prohibiting suicide and then quickly reimposed it, decreeing that failed suicides be imprisoned in the rapidly expanding state hospital system.[35] The psychiatric quackery that they legitimized as medical science and unleashed on the Western world has had a far-reaching influence on the modern perception of suicide as a manifestation of mental illness. The alienist Jean Etienne Dominique Esquirol (1772–1840)—who, along with Philippe Pinel (1745–1826), is considered the founder of French psychiatry—declared: "Onanism is . . . one of the causes of suicide. . . . Individuals thus enfeebled . . . form no other purpose than that of ridding themselves of life, which they have no longer the capacity to endure. . . . Insanity, or mental alienation, is a cerebral affection, ordinarily chronic, and without fever."[36] The belief that masturbation is pathogenic persisted well into the twentieth century; the belief that mental disease is brain disease is as popular today as it was in Esquirol's day.

Emil Kraepelin (1856–1926), the German psychiatrist who invented the first system of psychiatric classification, lent further credence to the doctrine that mental patients are dangerous to themselves and others. He wrote: "All the insane are dangerous, in some degree, to their neighbors, and even more so to themselves. . . . [A]ssaults, thefts, and impostures are often committed by those whose minds are diseased. . . . The treatment of the malady cannot, as a rule, be carried out, except in an asylum, as thoughts of suicide are almost always present."[37]

Along with the practice of excusing the successful suicide by means of a posthumous finding of not guilty by reason of insanity, nineteenth-century English law punished unsuccessful suicide, typically by hanging. In 1860, a Russian visitor named Nicholas Ogarev gave this account of such an occurrence:

A man was hanged who had cut his throat, but had been brought back to life. They hanged him for suicide. The doctor had warned them that it was impossible to hang him as the throat would burst open and he would breathe through the aperture. They did not listen to his advice and hanged their man. The wound immediately opened and the man came back to life again although he was hanged. . . . [T]hey bound up the neck below the wound until he died.[38]

It would be a mistake to believe that we long ago abandoned such a barbaric practice. Robert Brecheen, a resident of Oklahoma sentenced to death for murder, was scheduled to be executed by lethal injection at midnight on October 10, 1995. At 9 P.M. that night, the guards found him in a semicomatose state from "an overdose of sedatives. He was taken to a hospital, treated and revived. He was then returned to prison . . . where he was executed by injection."[39]

English criminal law continued to punish unsuccessful suicide until astonishingly recently. During the decade 1946–1955, about 5,000 persons who attempted suicide were brought to trial, and all but about 350 were found guilty; some were imprisoned, others were fined or put on probation. In 1955, "a sentence of two years' imprisonment was imposed on a man for trying to commit suicide in prison." On appeal, this sentence was reduced to one month's imprisonment.[40] As recently as 1969, a court on the Isle of Man "ordered an adolescent to be whipped for attempting suicide."[41] Not until the passage of the so-called Suicide Act in 1961 was unsuccessful suicide removed from English criminal law. Instead of simply repealing criminal penalties for unsuccessful suicide, the Act mandated that every unsuccessful suicide be examined by a psychiatrist.[42]

As long as the law categorized attempted suicide as a crime, society had to deal with the criminals the law created. When the public became dissatisfied with punishing failed suicides by executing them, the law extended the excuse of insanity to failed suicides, punishing them instead with deprivation of liberty in the insane asylum. In the United States, unsuccessful suicide is routinely "punished" by such sanctions. Jerome Motto, M.D., professor of psychiatry at the University of California in San Francisco, explains: "If the patient refuses voluntary ongoing treatment, involuntary measures would be indicated to the extent that the law permits."[43]

Modern Psychiatry and Suicide

The main bogeys of nineteenth-century psychiatrists were self-abuse and self-murder (masturbation and suicide). Both behaviors became the bogeys of the psychoanalysts as well. In 1910, Freud concluded the first essay in which he specifically addressed the subject of suicide with these words: "Let us suspend our judgment till experience has solved this problem."[44] What is the problem? It was "know[ing] how it becomes possible for the extraordinarily powerful life instinct to be overcome." In 1917, Freud announced his famous solution—self-murder is aggression turned against the self: "[N]o neurotic harbors thoughts of suicide which he has not turned back upon himself from murderous impulses against others."[45] Freud's sweeping generalization is a sobering reminder of the powerful influence of the religious-psychiatric tradition: He treats suicide as if it were a unitary phenomenon.

Carl Jung's (1875–1961) declared views on suicide were similar to those of his psychiatric colleagues. He maintained that killing oneself is wrong, legally as well as psychologically. But this was only a facade necessary to maintain his status as a psychiatrist. For many years, Jung kept "a loaded pistol next to his bed and vowed to blow his brains out if he ever felt he had entirely lost his sanity."[46] Nevertheless, when he was 76 years old, he wrote to a woman who had "attempted suicide": "You ought to realize that suicide is murder, since after suicide there remains a corpse exactly as with any ordinary murder. . . . That is the reason why the Common Law punishes a man that tries to commit suicide, and it is psychologically true too."[47] Fearing the loss of one's sanity is hardly a reason for keeping a pistol *next to one's bed*; and although disease, war, famine, and killing in self-defense all result in corpses, none is considered murder.

Psychiatrists have never had to and have never confronted the history of psychiatry. This is mainly why the public remains in impenetrable darkness about psychiatrists' mistakes and misdeeds and why their pronouncements continue to carry the weight of professional authority. Today, psychiatrists allege a causal connection between mental illness and suicide which, as I shall show, is a rich source of fresh psychiatric mistakes and misdeeds. Some examples of this unsupportable and unsupported contention follow:

> *The act [of suicide] clearly represents an illness and is, in fact, the least curable of all diseases.*
> —Ilza Veith, medical historian, 1969[48]

> *The contemporary physician sees suicide as a manifestation of emotional illness. Rarely does he view it in a context other than that of psychiatry.*
> —Editorial, Journal of the American Medical Association, 1967[49]

We are now also in agreement that this [suicide] is a public health matter and that the state should combat the disease of suicide.
— Stanley Yolles, director of the National Institute of Mental Health, 1967[50]

The idea that suicide is a manifestation and result of mental illness is attributable in part to the pervasive confusion, among lay persons and medical professionals alike, of diagnosis with disease. Most people now believe that if a particular behavior or state of mind—say, engaging in homosexual acts or feeling dejected—is authoritatively called a disease ("diagnosed"), then "it" is a disease, thereafter called a "diagnosable disease."* People also believe that (1) such a disease is the "cause" of the unwanted acts or feelings of the subject—who now becomes the patient; (2) the "patient" has no responsibility for his acts or feelings—now called "symptoms"; and (3) psychiatrists are authorized, perhaps even obligated, to treat the patient's disease with or without the patient's permission. The following statement by Herbert Hendin, executive director of the American Foundation for Suicide Prevention, and (the late) Gerald Klerman (professor of psychiatry at Columbia University) illustrates this view:

We know that 95% of those who kill themselves have been shown to have a diagnosable psychiatric illness in the months preceding suicide. The majority suffer from depression, which can be treated. . . . Other diagnoses among the suicides include alcoholism, substance abuse, schizophrenia, and panic disorders; treatments are available for all of these illnesses. . . . Given the advances in our medical knowledge and treatment ability thorough psychiatric evaluation for the presence of a treatable disorder may literally make the difference between choosing life or choosing death for patients. . . . This is not an evaluation that can be made by the average physician. . . . Our efforts should concentrate on providing treatment . . . and, in the case of terminal illness, helping the individual come to terms with death.[51]

Hendin and Klerman do not say who is choosing life or death: doctor or patient. They do not specify their criteria for determining whether a person has a "diagnosable psychiatric illness." Nor do they explain why a "diagnosable psychiatric illness" entitles the psychiatrist to treat the patient against his will. (Hendin and Klerman conflate the psychiatrist's [alleged] "treatment ability" with his access to the persons they propose to treat.)

The term "suicidology" deserves a brief remark in this connection. Coined in Germany (*Suicidologie*) in 1929, the term became popular after World War II, when its use was promoted by Edwin Shneidman, now pro-

---

*Conversely, most people believe that if a disease is authoritatively removed from the roster of official diagnoses, then it ceases to be a disease. Homosexuality is the most familiar example.

fessor of thanatology emeritus at the University of California at Los Angeles. He wrote: "It may well be that in light of current concepts and facts about human self-destruction a new (and more accurate) term may eventually come into general usage. . . . Suicidology is defined as the scientific study of suicidal phenomena."[52] That mask conceals its true goal, namely, the intention to medicalize voluntary death as an illness and justify coercive psychiatric suicide prevention (CPSP) as a life-saving treatment. The suicidologists' conclusions are embedded in their premise, namely, the conviction, in the words of the American Association of Suicidology, that "most suicidal persons desperately want to live."[53]

The view that suicide is a manifestation of mental illness is presented as if it were not only true but also beneficial for patient and public alike. This is not so. The interpretation is double-edged: It exonerates the actor from wrongdoing, but stigmatizes him as crazy; it justifies the psychiatrist's control of the patient, but makes him responsible for the patient's suicide. It is the psychiatrist's professional duty to commit the suicidal patient and treat him against his will. The nonmedical mental health professional—not (yet) licensed by the State to commit patients—must refer the patient to a psychiatrist. As a result, we cannot and do not judge suicide as we judge other morally freighted acts: as good or bad, desirable or undesirable, depending on the actor's circumstances and the observer's criteria. Instead, we explain away suicide by forming a confused concept that combines elements of sin, sickness, irrationality, incompetence, and insanity.

IS SUICIDE LEGAL?

If an act is legal—say, eating cereals for breakfast—then attempting to commit the act and assisting another to perform it are also legal. Conversely, if an act is illegal—say, murder—then attempting to commit the act and assisting another to perform it are also illegal. The prohibition of attempted and assisted suicide thus implies that suicide itself is illegal. Norman St. John-Stevas correctly observes: "If suicide itself is not a crime, then, theoretically, aiding and abetting it should not be either."[54] However, neither the Law nor society feels any need to be consistent in this matter.

Contemporary commentators routinely assert that suicide is "legal" and they often interpret this as evidence of our "liberation" from the uncivilized customs of the past. For example, a California court declared: "Suicide or attempted suicide is not a crime under the criminal statutes of California or any state. The absence of a criminal penalty for these acts is explained by the prevailing thought . . . that suicide or attempted suicide is an expression of mental illness that punishment cannot remedy."[55] Similarly, a spokesperson for the American Medical Association (AMA) asserted: "Since no penalty is attached to suicide in any state today (and probably could not be, due to constitutional prohibitions against forfeitures as punishment for crimes) ... therefore, without effective legal recognition of suicide [as a crime], the misdemeanor of attempted suicide cannot be legally created."[56]

However, the assertion that "suicide is legal" is true only *de jure*, in the narrowest meaning of the word "legal": There are no criminal penalties for successful suicide. *De facto*, suicide is not legal. Supreme Court Justice Antonin Scalia minced no words when he asserted that it is "absolutely plain that there is no right to die ... that the law had never countenanced suicide."[57] Justice Scalia's language reflects the conventional abhorrence of suicide. In the Anglo-American legal system, any act not prohibited by law is legal, although it may be immoral. For example, driving while intoxicated is illegal; however, getting drunk at home is legal, albeit it is not countenanced by law.

If suicide were legal, as divorce is legal, then the coercive prevention of suicide would be illegal: The psychiatrist who forcibly prevents a patient from killing himself would be considered a criminal, guilty of assault, battery, and kidnapping. This is not the case. Courts consistently affirm the opinion that suicide is the product of mental illness and that its coercive control is properly in the province of mental health law. Cheryl K. Smith, an attorney and one of the drafters of the 1994 Oregon Death with Dignity Act (DWDA), acknowledges: "While neither suicide nor attempted suicide are criminal acts in most states, a failed attempt at suicide may lead to involuntary psychiatric commitment. Under the laws in most states, a person who is a danger to self or others may be committed for evaluation."[58] Laws about suicide, explains legal scholar Ann Grace McCoy, are "predicated on the belief that there is no such thing as rational (legitimate or functional) suicide."[59] Most Americans realize that speaking about killing oneself (threatening suicide) and trying and failing to kill oneself (unsuccessful suicide) have very serious legal and social consequences, unlike threatening or failing to perform other legal acts. Moreover, transforming the religious dread of self-murder as a depravity into the medical dread of "suicide" as a disease and thus continuing to treat all acts of voluntary death as, *a priori*, wrongful also has very serious consequences. By treating all acts called "suicide" as tainted with insanity, we incapacitate ourselves from distinguishing between self-killing that we deem unjustifiable (due to free will or mental illness) and self-killing that we deem justifiable (due to discontinuing life-sustaining treatment).[60]

Suicide and the Rhetoric of Rights

Every living being dies. Death is a biological given, a fact. Right is a political construct, an attribute of *persons*. It is bad enough that we talk about a person's right to *refuse* medical treatment, instead of subsuming that supposed right under the crime of assault and battery for nonconsensual medical relations. It is even worse to talk about a person's right, as a terminally ill patient, to physician-assisted suicide—that is, to talk about a right that accrues to an individual by virtue of his being a victim (of dying slowly rather than quickly)—and thus create special legal privileges for *certain medically selected individuals (to obtain certain drugs or be killed by doctors).*

As long as suicide was called "self-murder," English-speaking people had no vocabulary with which to obscure the elemental fact that the self-killer engages in an act of deliberate, wrongful homicide. Today, in our politically and psychiatrically correct discourse about suicide, it is virtually impossible to express that opinion. We apply the legal-bureaucratic jargon of rights to both patients and doctors. If the patient is said to be suicidal, he has a "right to treatment"—and his physician has a right to treat him without his consent. If the patient is said to be terminally ill, he has a right to physician-assisted suicide—and his physician has a right to offer him death by prescription.

Anyone who values the Anglo-American tradition of civil rights must feel concerned about the prevailing political fashion of giving the members of certain groups—AIDS patients, heroin addicts, terminally ill persons—access to goods and services denied to everyone else and calling the exception for them a "right" and a "treatment." Instead of guaranteeing anyone's rights, this policy debases the very idea of rights.

Properly speaking, civil rights adhere to individuals as persons, not to individuals as members of one or another special group. That is why Anglo-American political philosophers have traditionally exempted the members of three groups of human beings from the class of full-fledged persons: the insane, idiots, and infants. Accordingly, children, retarded persons, and psychotics are considered unable to fulfill the social duties of normal adults (this is true for some and untrue for others), and individuals assigned to these categories are deprived of certain rights and exempted from certain responsibilities. Traditionally, deprivations of rights and responsibilities went hand in hand. Now the relationship is often inverted: Members of certain groups of "victims" are exempted from responsibilities the rest of us must shoulder, and are accorded rights of which the rest of us are deprived. This policy rests on the following reasoning. Substance S is an illegal drug: the State prohibits the sale, possession, and use of it. However, patient P suffers from disease D and will derive benefits from substance S. *Ergo*, patient P and the physician treating him ought to be exempted from the sanctions of our drug laws with respects to the prescription, possession, and use of substance S. Activists for medical marijuana, for methadone treatment, and for PAS agitate accordingly for dispensations for glaucoma patients, heroin addicts, and terminally ill patients and their physicians. Patients and doctors alike reject repealing the drug laws that would grant everyone his right to drugs.[61]

Defining suicide as a problem—a disease to be prevented and treated—radically limits our understanding of it and our options for responding to it soberly. The rule that every problem in life is also a solution, and vice versa, applies to suicide as well. Clearly, killing oneself is, *inter alia*, a protection from a fate considered worse than death. Furthermore, it is simply fallacious to attribute suicide to the subject's *present condition*, whether depression or any other illness or suffering. Killing oneself is a *future-directed, anticipatory act, an existential safety-net*. People save money not because they are indigent, but to prevent becoming indigent. People kill themselves not because they are suffering, but to prevent future suffering. Suicide is the emergency cord we want to be able to pull when we do not want to wait until the train stops at the station.

DESTIGMATIZING SELF-KILLING BY DENYING IT IS SUICIDE

When suicide was perceived as self-murder and was called by that name, it was reasonable to bracket it with murder. However, to still bracket suicide with murder, as if the two phenomena belonged in the same class, is as absurd as bracketing rape with consensual sexual relations. We also bracket suicide with accident, as a type of "unnatural death"; this is as absurd as bracketing philanthropy with theft. Suicide, like philanthropy, is, par excellence, wanted and willed by the subject; theft, like accident, is unwanted and unwilled by the subject. Linguistically, a "willed accident" is an oxymoron; it is properly called a "fake accident," which, if used to defraud an insurance company, is a crime. *Mutatis mutandis*, an "unwilled suicide," is also an oxymoron; it is properly called a "fake suicide," which, if used to cover up a murder, is also a crime. This does not mean that a person cannot kill himself by accident; indeed he can, for example by falling and suffering a fatal head injury. However, we call that "accidental death" not "accidental suicide."

A brief remark about the concept of unnatural death is in order here. Although there is obviously nothing literally unnatural about any death, journalists, health statisticians, politicians, and physicians still routinely refer to murder, suicide, and accident as "unnatural deaths," as opposed to "natural deaths" from diseases and injuries. This is a semantic subterfuge for making a different kind of distinction, namely, between death from a *medically undesirable* cause (such as disease) and death from a *morally undesirable* cause (such as murder). When the term "unnatural"—long applied to disapproved sexual acts—is applied to suicide, its function is to condemn it as an act that, regardless of circumstances, is "abnormal."

As long as we view suicide as unnatural—that is, wrongful—we must *blame* someone or something for it; for example, the devil, insanity, songs, television shows, and so forth.[62] The great religious reformers Martin Luther and John Calvin believed that suicide "was the work of the devil."[63] The great transformers of morality into medicine, the mental health professionals, believe that suicide is the work of bad songs, bad television shows, and other bad social influences—resulting in mental illnesses that cause people, especially young people, to kill themselves. Enlightened by such scientific information, in 1997 the father of a son who committed suicide told a Senate committee that the music Antichrist Superstar "caused him to kill himself."[64]

Before we can destigmatize suicide—assuming that is what we want to do—we must acknowledge that killing oneself is still an intensely stigmatized act. Instead of being stigmatized by religion, it is now stigmatized by medicine (psychiatry): Conventional wisdom and the media routinely attribute suicide to mental illness; the law accepts a psychiatric imputation of suicidality as a justification for depriving the subject of liberty and calling his imprisonment "hospitalization"; and Jewish and Christian clergymen accept the equation of suicide and insanity as a justification for evading the religious penalties for taking one's own life.

Probably because few people are willing to acknowledge these prejudices and practices, most intellectuals and scholars who address the subject of suicide—perhaps especially bioethicists—prefer to destigmatize the act by denying its very nature: they call instances or types of self-killing of which they approve—for example discontinuing hemodialysis and physician-assisted suicide—"not suicide." However, history teaches us that this gambit is doomed to failure.

The collective tainting of behaviors or persons cannot be ameliorated, much less abolished, by manipulating the vocabulary used for debasing them. The stigmatization of Jews in Christendom was not abolished by their religious conversion. The stigmatization of homosexuality was not abolished by its classification as an illness. Indeed, such maneuvers subtly legitimize the stigma and perpetuate the social attitudes they ostensibly try to alter. Nevertheless, medical professionals, the media, and the public are intensifying their efforts to destigmatize suicide by medicalizing every aspect of voluntary death.

In the years following World War II, it became fashionable to assert that we, Americans, "deny death." This is not true. We do not deny death; we are obsessed with it. We deny suicide by attributing its cause to nearly everything—from rock music to natural disasters and, above all else, to mental illness—except the subject's own decision. We are willing to *accuse* people and drugs and songs and TV shows of causing suicide; we are willing to *ex-*

cuse suicide by blaming it on several of the causes listed and, above all, on mental illness; but we are not willing to *accept* suicide as suicide.

When, but a century ago, infant mortality was high and death was commonplace, people worried not about dying, but about living and being punished in the hereafter. Today, when infant mortality is low, life expectancy is nearly four score, and most people never see a dead body, people worry about when and how they will die. Our fearful fascination with death is so intense and so indiscriminate that we dread not only the prospect of being killed by disease, but also the possibility of killing ourselves—a choice we have converted into the concern of "being killed" by mental illness.

Manipulating the Meaning of Suicide: Self-Killing as Not Suicide

The belief that our life on earth is only a prelude to a more fully realized life after death, that death is a door through which we pass in order to enter a better or truer life, is a theme basic to Christianity as well as to Islam. It is only a short step from defining death as rebirth to defining self-killing as not suicide. The simplest way to deny that a particular act or type of voluntary death is suicide is to manipulate the vocabulary—calling suicide *not suicide*, a tactic that, as I suggested, is similar to denying that a Jew is a Jew by calling him a Christian. Here are two examples.

In 1997, 39 persons in California, identified as members of a group called "Heaven's Gate," killed themselves. After their deaths we learned that the group's Web site featured an antisuicide statement, titled "Our Position Against Suicide," which set forth the following explanation for their mass suicide: "In these last days we are focused on . . . making a last attempt at telling the truth about how the Next Level may be entered (our last effort at offering to individuals of this civilization the way to avoid 'suicide')."[65]

A few weeks later, the Associated Press featured the story of the death of Father Dom Christian de Cherge, the leader of a group of French Trappist monks who chose to live among hostile Muslims in Algeria. The rebels announced that they would kill the monks if they did not leave. Vowing to stay, Father Dom Christian wrote: "My death, clearly, will appear to justify those who hastily judged me naive or idealistic. . . . But these people must realize that my most avid curiosity will then be satisfied. For then I shall be able, if God wills it, to immerse my gaze in that of the Father, and contemplate with him his Islamic children just as he sees them, all shining with the glory of Christ."[66]

In the case of Heaven's Gate, a collectivity quickly branded and dismissed as a "cult," the members classified their voluntary death as not suicide, but the media and the public viewed it as suicide. In the case of Father Dom Christian, a respected Catholic priest, the subject viewed his indirect self-killing as love of God, and the media and the public accepted it as a kind of martyrdom.

Now I want to consider the denial of a quite different kind of motive for suicide (or threating suicide), namely, blackmail. Because every attachment to another human being carries with it the potential of loss, it is a potential source of extortion or blackmail. If John loves Mary, Mary can try to extort certain concessions from John by threatening to leave him. The ultimate act of leaving another is killing oneself. Threats of suicide by adolescents and young people rejected by their lovers are often so motivated—the blackmailer trying to extort from parents or partners more compliant behavior or at least feelings of guilt.[67] Although we are more familiar with this strategy when the blackmailer threatens another person rather than himself—for example, a terrorist trying to extort money or other concessions by threatening to do violence to hostages—blackmail is more often the motive for autohomicide than it is for heterohomicide.

Nevertheless, even when it is obvious that a person threatens to kill himself to control the behavior of others, the pressure to attribute suicide to mental illness makes us unable to see that the motive for it is blackmail. (Unsuccessful blackmail is still blackmail.) The following vignette is an example. On February 20, 1998, the police in Lexington, Kentucky, were dispatched to the Jones's home to serve an arrest warrant for Bob Jones, a.k.a. Bob Higgins, a once-famous black activist and fugitive from the law. When Jones opened the door and realized that the callers were policemen who came to arrest him, he slammed it shut, "ran to the rear of the house and reappeared, holding two knives to his throat. 'Don't come in,' he screamed. 'I'll kill myself if you come in.' " His wife Gayl, a prominent black writer, also threatened to kill herself "if the police stormed the house." The police stormed the house. Bob Jones fatally stabbed himself. Gayl Jones was committed to the state mental hospital.[68]

The determination to destigmatize suicide by attributing it to forces outside the subject leads us to stubbornly misinterpret all contrary evidence. As recently as mid-century, if a person who killed himself left a suicide note, it was accepted as proof that his death was due to suicide. This is no longer true. Regardless of the evidence, what counts as suicide is now defined by the psychiatrically informed expert, as the following example illustrates. A 17-year-old boy leaps to his death in a Syracuse (New York) shopping mall, the same spot from which a young woman had jumped to her death a few weeks earlier. The medical examiner dismisses the boy's suicide note, stating: "[H]e was so high on drugs that . . . he did not understand the 'lethality' of his actions."[69]

Finally, contemporary tactics to destigmatize suicide by taking literally the pretense that it is caused by an amoral disease are leading us to exonerate persons convicted of crimes. On June 28, 1998, Slavko Dokmanovic, the ex-Mayor of Vukovar in Croatia convicted of war crimes, hanged himself in his cell. Sentencing was scheduled for July 7. The defendant was said to have been "on medication for depression." The United Nations War Crimes Tribunal in The Hague ended the proceedings. A spokesperson explained: "There will be no verdict now and the case is herewith terminated."[70] The suicides of leading Nazis were not interpreted as exculpatory evidence. Herman Goering's suicide during the Nuremberg trials in 1946 had no impact on the court proceedings, and no one construed it as annulling his guilt. Suicide has not changed since then. *We have changed.* We regard the person who kills himself—regardless of his (mis)deeds—as a victim.

The claim that untreated mental illness causes suicide can, of course, be easily turned upside down into the claim that the *treatment of mental illness* causes suicide. In the present climate of tort litigation, large companies are ideal targets for legal blackmail. Not surprisingly, psychiatrists who exalt the drug treatment of mental illness claim that depression causes suicide, while psychiatrists who execrate such treatment claim that psychiatric drugs cause suicide.[71] Both sets of claimants champion self-serving lies. Neither psychosis nor Prozac causes suicide.[72] Tragic, threatening, unhappy life events may make a person consider and perhaps choose suicide as a way out of his dilemma. But they do not *cause* suicide. Every day countless persons are the victims of a host of misfortunes. Most endure their fate. Only a small minority kill themselves. In the final analysis, killing oneself is *always a choice.*

Interpreting Suicide: *Cui Bono*?[73]*

Ironically, the people who most earnestly deny that suicide is "natural"—in the sense that it is an understandable, reasonable choice given the subject's situation and mind set—are the very persons whose job it is to deal with conflicts sometimes resolved by suicide: namely, psychiatrists, politicians, and lawyers. To be sure, each of these professionals deals with conflicts that affect others, not himself: the psychiatrist, with conflicts that affect patients; the politician, with conflicts among groups and nations; the lawyer, with conflicts between plaintiffs and defendants. Although this is troubling stuff, it is also comforting: Other people's troubles help to divert

---

*This rhetorical question, intended to make explicit the hidden interests of parties to a conflict, was popularized by Cicero, who attributed it to a Roman judge. Cicero wrote: "When trying a case, the famous judge L. Cassius never failed to inquire, 'Who gained by it?' [*Cui bono?*]. Man's character is such that no one undertakes crimes without hope of gain."

the professional's attention from his own. When the conflict takes place on the professional's own turf—within himself or in his own family—then he often behaves even more cowardly than do ordinary people.

We often believe what we *know* is not true because, if we did not believe it, we would be compelled to change our behavior, relinquish our false beliefs, and forgo benefits to which we have become accustomed. Asked whether he believed President Clinton's January 1998 declaration that he did not have sex with Monica Lewinsky, Erskine B. Bowles, then White House chief of staff, offered this candid reply: "If I didn't believe him, I couldn't stay. So I believed him."[74] People often attribute suicide to depression for the same reason.

In July 1995, Vincent W. Foster, Jr., deputy White House counsel, was found dead in a suburban Washington, DC park, with a bullet through his head. The official cause of death was suicide. A few weeks before his death, Foster had written a memo in which he described Whitewater as "a can of worms you shouldn't open."[75] Evidently deciding that her husband's political entanglements had nothing to do with his suicide, Lisa Foster began to see a psychiatrist and take Prozac: "The antidepressant," explained Peter J. Boyer in *The New Yorker*, "gave her an understanding, for the first time, of Vince and his illness. 'That's when I realized that it was a disease,' she says. . . . Lack of serotonin. . . . Lisa has found some solace in the diagnosis of depression." Quoted in the same article Laura Foster, her daughter, says, "It's a whole lot easier seeing him as sick and having a chemical imbalance than to feel 'Oh, my God, he did this and he knew what he was doing.' It's easier to say it wasn't his fault."

When AIDS or cancer kills a person by destroying his vital functions, his relatives deplore the disease. When mental illness "kills" a person by suicide, his "loved ones" rejoice in the diagnosis. *Cui bono?* As we approach the end of the century, the medicalization of suicide is as complete as the medicalization of masturbation was at the beginning of the century. It is obvious that any interpretation of suicide in general—for example, that it *is* a sin or a crime or a sign of mental illness or aggression turned against the self or a free choice—is bound to be false. Suicide may be—may "mean"—almost anything.

We should neither abhor nor admire a death merely because it is voluntary. Instead, we should distinguish among the great variety of circumstances in which people kill themselves and the many reasons why they do so. And we should accept death control as a personal choice and responsibility, just as we accept birth control as a personal choice and responsibility. In short, our laws and medical practices should neither hinder nor facilitate suicide.

Excusing Suicide

The Fateful Evasion

Reluctance to punish when punishment is needed seems to me not benevolence but cowardice, and I think that the proper attitude of mind toward criminals is not long-suffering charity but open enmity; for the object of the criminal law is to overcome evil with evil.

—Sir James Fitzjames Stephen (1829–1894)[1]

Lies are the mortar that binds the savage individual man into the social masonry.

—H. G. Wells (1866–1946)[2]

We speak not in order to say something, but in order to obtain a particular effect.

—Josef Goebbels (1897–1945)[3]

In the Christian world view, human life is God's gift and property. Hence, suicide is self-murder, *felo de se* (felony against oneself). Inasmuch as the legitimacy of the Christian sovereign's rule rested on his special relationship to God, self-murder was also an offense against him and was accordingly punished by both canon and criminal law.

With suicide defined as a species of murder, the persons sitting in judgment of self-killers had the duty to punish them. Since punishing suicide required doing injustice to innocent parties, in particular to the minor children of the deceased, eventually the task proved to be an intolerable burden. In the seventeenth century, men sitting on coroners' juries began to recoil against desecrating the corpse and dispossessing the suicide's dependents of their means of support. However, their religious beliefs precluded repealing the laws punishing the crime. Their only recourse was to evade the laws: The doctrine that the self-killer is *non compos mentis* and hence not responsible for his act accomplished this task.

The transformation of *self-killing from a deliberate act* into the *unintended consequence of a disease (of the mind-brain)* forms the foundation of the pseudoscience of psychiatry and the vastly influential institutions of social control that rest on its claims called "theories" and coercions called "treatments." The "insanitizing of suicide" precedes the birth of psychiatry. Psychiatry is the result, not the cause, of the transformation of self-murder from sin-and-crime into illness-as-excuse.

A BRIEF HISTORY OF THE DEFENSE AGAINST SUICIDE

The impetus for excusing self-murder did not come from its ostensible beneficiary, the victim of the law against suicide. Indeed, it could not come from him: The suicide was dead; his family, bereft of means and reputation, was powerless. Instead, the impetus came from those who needed the "reform" and had the political clout to bring it about: the coroners and coroners' juries who sought to evade the burden of having to impose harsh penalties on the corpses of suicides and the widows and children they left behind.

The practice of routinely excusing self-killers as insane led, inevitably, to preventing suicide by incarcerating potential self-killers in insane asylums. That practice, in turn, reinforced the belief that persons who kill themselves are insane, that the insane are likely to kill themselves, and that "being dangerous to oneself (and to others)" justifies depriving people of liberty. For three hundred years, the legal and medical justification for psychiatric preventive detention (civil commitment) has rested comfortably and securely on that set of beliefs.

Melancholia: Laying the Ground for Excusing Self-Murder

The earliest English text linking suicide to what psychiatrists today call "clinical depression" is *The Anatomy of Melancholy* (1621), by Robert Burton (1577–1640), an Anglican minister who became a madhouse keeper.[4]* Distressed by both suicide and the penalties against it, Burton lamented: "After many tedious dayes at last, either by drowning, hanging or some such fearful end, they precipitate, or make away with themselves. . . . 'Tis a common calamity, a fatal end to this *disease*, they are condemned to a violent

---

*I use the terms "melancholia," "depression," and "clinical depression" interchangeably. The adjective "clinical" is purely instrumental: Its function is to separate normal sorrow from an ostensibly pathological condition that justifies (involuntary) psychiatric intervention.

death . . . if that *heavenly Physician*, by his assisting grace and mercy alone do not prevent."[5]

Burton's language is religious, not medical. It would be a mistake to interpret his use of the term "melancholy" as denoting a disease in our own modern materialist sense, a concept that did not exist in the seventeenth century. When Burton used the term "melancholy," he had in mind a Galenic malady, that is, an ailment believed to be a manifestation of humoral imbalance affecting not only the brain but also "The Heart . . . as Melanelius proves out of Galen . . . and the Midriffe, and many other parts."[6] The prevention of this "disease" lay in the hands of Jesus, whom Burton appropriately calls "the heavenly Physician."

The importance of Burton's work is legal, religious, and social, not medical: He articulated the basis for the insanity defense against self-murder and, derivatively, against murder. Burton did not deny that suicide was a mortal sin and a capital crime. Nor did he claim to possess novel medical information. He merely pleaded, with God and his Sovereign, for relaxing the punishment of melancholiacs who kill themselves: Their penalty ought to "be mitigated, as in such as are mad . . . or found to have been long melancholy . . . they know not what they do, deprived of reason . . . as in a ship that is void of a Pilot . . . [destined to] suffer shipwreck. . . . We ought not to be so rash and rigorous in our censures, as some are . . . God be merciful unto us all."[7]

How could the law against suicide temper justice with mercy? The only way it could do so was by transforming the self-killer from a responsible person (moral agent) into an inanimate object (a pilotless ship tossed about by a raging sea). That is precisely what the psychiatrization of the law against suicide has done: It *recast self-killing from a deliberate felony into a purposeless accident (or medical negligence)*. Burton's plea presages the posthumous diagnosis of the self-murderer as insane or *non compos mentis*, hence not responsible for killing himself. Once the principle was established that a post-crime diagnosis of mental illness excuses self-murder, it was logical to extend it to excusing murder and, potentially, any other crime. These extensions are enshrined in the so-called McNaghten and Durham Rules.[8]

Burton's treatise on melancholia was emblematic of seventeenth-century works that sought to mitigate the rigors of the antisuicide laws by transforming badness into madness. John Sym (1581–1637), also a clergyman, pleaded for mercy for the self-killer and his family, arguing that the "motive occasioning self-killing is phrentick distemperatures. . . . [A]lthough all self-murderers are self-killers, yet all self-killers are not self-murderers."[9] Sym too believed in the humoral theory of disease and acknowledged that killing oneself is both a sin and a crime. He asked only that the lunatic self-killer be spared the harsh punishment that the laws of England prescribed for him.

In 1672, Gideon Harvey, physician to King Charles II, published a treatise bearing the remarkable title, *Morbus Anglicus*, a term he used partly to identify "hypochondriacal melancholy" as a specific disease, and partly to propose the novel medical theory that this disease had a special affinity for Englishmen, a notion that proved popular among them.[10] With George Cheyne's publication of his classic *The English Malady* in 1733, this canard became a fact. What sorts of conditions did Cheyne have in mind when he spoke of the English Malady? Ailments such as "Hysterical Distemper," "Lowness of Spirits, "Spleen," and "Vapours," each condition supposedly treatable with mercury, antimony, and other arcane compounds and concoctions.[11]

In 1600, there were no mental hospitals, as we know them. By 1700, there was a flourishing new industry called the "trade in lunacy."[12] I have described elsewhere the social circumstances and forces that contributed to the creation of this forerunner of the nineteenth-century insane asylum and the twentieth-century mental hospital.[13] Here I want to comment briefly on one of these forces, the insanitizing of suicide.

Insanitizing Suicide: Medicalizing Mercy

The Latin word *compos* means controlled, as in *compos mentis* (controlled mind or sane). For centuries, the term *non compos mentis* was used narrowly, to identify individuals incapable of caring for themselves and to justify appointing guardians over them. Rarely was the phrase used as an excuse for crime, and then only in cases of murder, to reduce the penalty from execution to life imprisonment. In the late Middle Ages, the frequency of suicide in England increased dramatically and, in tandem with it, so did the excuse of *non compos mentis* to evade the penalty for it.

The view that suicide is wrongful is, as we have seen, of ancient origin. In England, the deed was formally condemned in A.D. 673 by the Council of Hereford. At first, the penalty was denial of burial rites; then it became the practice to bury the corpse at the crossroads, with a stake driven through the body; in the tenth century, forfeiting the suicide's property and bestowing it on the sovereign's Almoner was added.* Here is what the celebrated

---

*We view the practice of punishing suicide with the forfeiture of the deceased man's property, penalizing his innocent family, as barbaric, yet we view the practice of treating suicidality with the forfeiture of the would-be suicide's liberty as enlightened. This runs counter to the principle of punishing crimes in proportion to their severity, from deprivation of property (fine) as the least severe punishment, followed by deprivation of liberty (imprisonment), and deprivation of life (execution).

English jurist William Blackstone (1723–1780) had to say about these practices:

The law of England wisely and religiously considers that no man has the power to
destroy life, but by commission from God, the author of it; and as the suicide is
guilty of a double offence, one spiritual, in evading the prerogative of the Almighty,
and rushing into His immediate presence uncalled for, the other temporal, against
the sovereign, who has an interest in the preservation of all his subjects, the law has
therefore ranked this among the highest crimes, making it a peculiar species of felony committed on one's self.[14]

Blackstone recognized the subterfuge and warned against it: "But this
excuse [of finding the offender to be *non compos mentis*] ought not to be
strained to the length to which our coroner's juries are apt to carry it, viz.,
that every act of suicide is an evidence of insanity; as if every man who acts
contrary to reason had no reason at all; for the same argument would prove
every other criminal *non compos*, as well as the self-murderer."[15]*

It was a futile warning: The law itself *defined the jury's posthumous "diagnosis" of the dead man's "mind" as an instance of genuine fact finding.* People
need no encouragement to evade responsibility. Yet, here, the Law, the
Great Teacher, invited just such an evasion. By declaring suicides *non compos mentis*, the Law had crafted a mechanism for rejecting responsibility
and, aided by the medical profession, wrapped the deception and self-
deception in the mantle of healing and science.

Why did the insanity defense against self-murder develop when it did
and where it did? The answer lies in the rapid economic development of
England in the seventeenth century and the accompanying spread of culture and social sensibility. It was this—not melancholy—that was a novel
feature of the English social landscape: For the first time in history, people
at large, not just a few philosophers, began to take seriously the twin ideas
of personal liberty and right to property. One result, as noted already, was
that men sitting on coroners' juries found it increasingly more difficult to
deprive innocent wives and children of their dead husband's possessions.
But the jurors were in a bind. Repealing the laws against self-murder was
politically unthinkable, yet punishing the deed as prescribed by law was
morally unacceptable.

There is an important similarity here between the dilemma of punishing
self-homicide (suicide) then and punishing abortion (feticide) today. Both
acts entail the deliberate taking of human life (homicide). Both may be
treated as crimes. In the climate of our modern popular opinion, both acts

---

*English laws mandating that the suicide be buried at the crossroads and his property be con-
fiscated were repealed only in 1823 and 1870, respectively.

are practically unpunishable. Rational criminal sanctions against abortion would require punishing the agent, the pregnant woman, more severely than her deputy, the abortionist. Rational criminal sanctions against suicide, absent an alliance between Church and State or Medicine and State, is a contradiction in terms.

In eighteenth-century England, the solution to the dilemma of punishing self-murder as prescribed by law was to treat the person guilty of the crime as if he were a lunatic—a tactic I call "insanitizing suicide." This maneuver allowed society to condemn self-killing as a moral and legal offense, to maintain the religious and legal sanctions against it, and to provide a seemingly enlightened mechanism for not punishing the act as required by law. S. E. Sprott, a historian of eighteenth-century English suicide, remarks: "Juries increasingly brought in findings of insanity *in order* to save the family from the consequences of a verdict of felony; the number of deaths recorded as 'lunatic' grew startlingly in relation to the number recorded as self-murder. . . . [B]y the 1760s confiscation of goods seems to have become rare."[16] It must have been clear to anyone who gave thought to the matter that finding the suicide's "mind" *non compos*—posthumously, exactly at the moment when he was executing his felonious deed—was a *semantic-legal strategy* for circumventing the penalty the law prescribed for this crime.

Faced with tough choices about delicate matters, people often prefer evasion to confrontation. The social utility, perhaps necessity, of not facing up to the moral challenge that suicide poses for us is dramatically illustrated by the death of Robert Stewart Londonderry, better known as Viscount Castlereagh (1769–1822). Believing, probably correctly, that he was being blackmailed for homosexual acts, Castlereagh, who had served as both secretary of war and foreign secretary, slashed his throat and was buried, in a ceremony befitting his station, at Westminster Abbey.[17] Nevertheless, the instrumental-tactical character of this policy has remained officially unacknowledged, perhaps even unrecognized, to this day.

The Insanity Excuse: *Cui Bono?*

Blackstone feared that excusing dead self-murderers as insane would lead to also excusing living murderers and other criminals as insane, thus defeating *the very purpose of the criminal law, namely, meting out punishment.* In large measure, that has come to pass. But there was worse to come. Blackstone did not anticipate that there was a far greater danger lurking in the insanity excuse—that the State might one day find it convenient to attribute insanity not only to criminals but to noncriminals as well, subjecting both groups to *de facto* imprisonment under the guise of treatment. This, too, has come to pass: We now live, as I have suggested, in a Therapeutic State.[18]

Blackstone could not have anticipated this development, which depends on a perversion of the concept of excuse. In legal tradition, an excuse for a crime is a condition that absolves the actor of what, in its absence, would be an offense against the Law; for example, self-defense is an "excusing condition" against assault and murder. The person so excused goes free. The person excused on the ground of insanity goes to an insane asylum.

Furthermore, it is an ancient and uncontested legal principle that ignorance of the law is *not* an excusing condition in law. "Ignorance of those things which one is bound to know excuses not," said Sir Matthew Hale (1609–1676), Lord Chief Justice under Charles II. This maxim is an essential principle of the criminal law because, as *Black's Law Dictionary* explains: "Every man must be taken to be cognizant of the law; otherwise there is no saying to what extent the excuse of ignorance may not be carried."[19] The point is obvious: The person who successfully pleads an "excusing condition" to a crime (except insanity) is excused as not guilty of it. The law can no more lay a hand on him than it can lay a hand on any person not accused or convicted of a felony. This is why criminal defendants use every possible excuse available to them: They have nothing to fear from pleading it successfully. Conversely, this is why prosecutors never attribute an excuse to a criminal defendant: They have nothing to gain from doing so.

With insanity as a defense, the incentives are inverted. The defendant who successfully pleads mental illness is invalidated as a mental patient and is incarcerated in a mental hospital. Exactly the same thing happens to the defendant to whom his adversaries—prosecutor, jury, judge—successfully attribute a defense of insanity. That is why prosecutors and defense attorneys, especially if appointed by the court or the defendant's relatives, often seek to impose an insanity defense on the accused, even against his express wishes.[20*]

To understand the far-reaching significance of the expansion, during the past two centuries, not just of the reality but also of the *legitimacy of state power masquerading as medical diagnosis and treatment*, we need to reconsider briefly the historical grounds for the legitimacy of the State in English and American political thought.

Life is full of dangers, mainly of two types, natural and human. Earthquakes and floods are instances of dangers from the natural environment; theft, assault, and murder are instances of dangers from the human environment. From Hobbes and Locke to the Framers of the Constitution, political philosophers have agreed that the principal (or only) moral justification for the State, as a political entity with a monopoly over the

---

*This is most likely to happen to defendants charged with crimes considered abhorrent, such as John W. Hinckley, Jr.

rightful use of force, is the protection of people from injury at the hands of other people, criminals at home and enemies abroad. In other words, the legitimacy of the state rests on a tacit understanding ("compact"): In exchange for our renouncing, as private persons, the use of force in relation to our fellow man, the State protects us from theft, assault, and murder.

The proposition that the self-killer, as lunatic, is a danger to himself from which he needs the coercive protection of the State violates this core principle. Evading the penalty for self-murder by insanitizing the deed legitimizes the fiction of a self divided against itself and, derivatively, the idea of insanity that entails the idea of "dangerousness to self and others" and the psychiatric edifice built on these ideas. Thus arose the belief and social practice that it is the duty of the State to protect, by force, insane persons from themselves (and others from insane persons as quasi-criminals). The result is a radical expansion of the authority, legitimacy, and power of the State—from using force to protect people from others to using force to protect people from themselves.

The truth about "insanity" is a good deal less sensational. Instead of a struggle in the soul between God and Satan or in the mind between sanity and insanity, the fact is that we all harbor diverse desires, some at odds with others. But we have only one self per person. The force of the maxim "actions speak louder than words" lies in its insistence that we not separate actor and action. The central task of the psychiatric excuse-makers is to destroy that unity by creating the fiction of insanity as a disease characterized by two (or more) selves, at war with one another.

Why did people adopt this belief in "mental illness"? Why does modern American society find the belief in "insanity" indispensable? Briefly, because the idea of insanity shields us from having to convict and execute certain offenders as prescribed by law: It gives us the option to excuse them as "not guilty by reason of insanity" and imprison them in mental hospitals (the insanity defense and insanity disposition). It also enables us to restrain certain troublesome persons (especially in the family) who would be difficult or impossible to control by means of criminal sanctions (civil commitment).[21]

THE BIRTH OF PSYCHIATRY: AUTO- AND HETEROHOMICIDE AS MADNESS

For centuries, the European mind, steeped in Christianity, treated murder and self-murder as two species of criminal homicides. It is not surprising, then, that excusing suicide by attributing it to insanity opened the door to excusing murder as well by attributing it to insanity. Before long, it became culturally plausible to blame all manner of socially offensive and undesirable behaviors on insanity. This characteristically modern dehumanization of man in the name of humanity is one of the poisoned fruits of the Enlightenment and of the French Revolution. All of the founders of psychiatry have contributed to its development, but perhaps none as much as did the acknowledged father of British psychiatry, Sir Henry Maudsley (1835–1918).

Sir Henry Maudsley

Maudsley did not invent the doctrine that the self-killer is insane, that his deed ought not be punished, and that anyone who wants to kill himself ought to be incarcerated in insane asylums. His claim to fame rests on popularizing it more effectively, at least in the English-speaking world, than did anyone else before him. Specifically, Maudsley secured the imprimatur of English Law and Medicine for the notion of "dangerousness to self and others" as a legitimate medico-legal concept and justification for the twin legal maneuvers of the insanity defense and involuntary mental hospitalization. By successfully insanitizing both self-murder and murder, Maudsley paradoxically reaccredited the seemingly discredited religious equation of the two acts. The Church maintained that the self-murderer, like the murderer, takes a life that belongs to God. Enlightenment philosophers successfully repudiated the belief that support this view; namely, that every living creature is God's property and, derivatively, that every subject is the property of the sovereign. Modern political philosophers tried to replace this religious-feudal construction of man's relation to authority with a secular-capitalist construction of it, recasting each person as his own master. This ambitious view rests on society's assumption that each person can be, wants to be, and is expected to be self-governing. Post-Enlightenment man's failure to live up to this expectation generated a reaction against the notion of personal self-ownership, epitomized by the ostensibly liberalizing psychiatric strategy of insanitizing suicide. Psychiatry has successfully refeudalized human life: It has turned Health into a property of Medicine and the Physician, much as Man had been the property of the Church and the Priest. Once again, suicide and murder are united as members of the same class; both cease to be perceived as motivated, intentional acts; both are reconstructed as the unintended consequences of uncontrollable "insane impulses." This interpretation, presented as medical discovery and "fact," was the foundation upon which Maudsley erected the empire of psychiatry, with life-saving suicide prevention as its principal mandate. He declared:

It is ... from the gloomy depths of a mind in this melancholic state that desperate impulses to suicide or homicide often spring. ... I do not see, therefore, how it can be justly maintained that an insane person should be subjected to any sort of punishment. . . . *The most anxious cases with which those have to do who are engaged in the care and treatment of the insane, are unquestionably those in which there is a persistent suicidal impulse . . . without appreciable disorder of the intellect.*[22]

Seemingly sane persons who want to kill themselves are, in fact, insane. Citing the case of a man confined in an insane asylum, Maudsley lamented that "one morning [he] eluded the vigilance of his attendants, ran off as fast as he could across hedges and ditches, closely but vainly pursued, to a railway, clambered up a high embankment, and deliberately laid himself down across the rails in front of a passing train, which killed him on the spot. Except that this unfortunate gentleman had the *insane suicidal impulse . . . he was in all respects apparently sane.*"[23]

Maudsley believed, and persuaded many others to believe, that the attribution of suicidality to a person by a psychiatrist is all the evidence the Law should require to establish that the person so "diagnosed" is insane; that such a person's intent is not his own and does not count as intent at all; and that the psychiatrist who incarcerates him in a mental hospital does not deprive him of liberty but saves his life. This set of beliefs now dominates the popular mind even more firmly than it did in Maudsley's day.

The reasons for the popularity of this doctrine lie buried deep in the heart of modern man. At its core lies a rejection of sober judgment and the duty to punish misbehavior unfailingly but fairly. As every parent knows, it is unpleasant to punish a child, especially one's own. Yet punishing him is a duty no less important than loving him and caring for him. Telling the child "it hurts me more than it hurts you" may sound sanctimonious, but it is nonetheless often true. Punishing an adult, especially if the penalty is severe, is also unpleasant: It places an existential burden on the shoulders of the punisher, greater in proportion as the punisher puts himself in the shoes of the punished. This is why people in modern mass societies—capitalist and socialist alike—prefer to control offenders with sanctions defined as therapeutic rather than those defined as punitive. For example, Karl Menninger (1893–1990), the dean of postwar American psychiatry, stated: "The principle of no punishment cannot allow any exception; it must apply in every case, even the worst case, the most horrible case, the most dreadful case—not merely the accidental, sympathy-arousing case."[24] Tomas Borge, Minister of the Interior of the Sandinista National Liberation Front, asserted: "There is a correspondence between Christian morals and our revolutionary morals. We both believe love is the fundamental element in the relations between men. . . . State coercion is an act of love."[25] Coercion, consecrated as love, is the ground on which religion, politics, and psychiatry meet and merge in the Therapeutic State.

It was easy to see through the Communists' claim that state coercion is an act of love; yet millions have let themselves be seduced by the siren song of therapeutic politics. It is just as easy to see through the psychiatrist's claim that therapeutic coercion is an act of love; yet millions have let themselves be seduced by the siren song of therapeutic justice. In reality, the "therapeutic attitude" is a woeful charade whose main function is to shield society—especially politicians, judges, and juries—from taking crime seriously and punishing lawbreakers in proportion to the gravity of their offenses. This societal impulse to reject the existential demands of punishing offenders, especially for serious crimes, is dramatically displayed in the historic case of Daniel McNaghten.[26]

The McNaghten Nontrial

On January 20, 1843, Daniel McNaghten, believing himself to be a "victim of the Tories," sought revenge by killing Sir Robert Peel, the Home Secretary. However, McNaghten mistook Edward Drummond, Peel's private secretary, for his boss, and killed him instead. There was no doubt that McNaghten had planned to kill Peel and had killed Drummond. McNaghten himself admitted to that. The trial began on February 2, 1843, with the Lord Chief Justice, Lord Abinger, asking McNaghten to plead: "How say you, prisoner, are you guilty or not guilty?" After a pause, McNaghten answered: "I am guilty of firing." Lord Abinger replied: "By that, do you mean to say you are not guilty of the remainder of the charge; that is, of intending to murder Mr. Drummond?" "Yes," replied McNaghten.[27]

Lord Abinger's phrasing of his question was legalistic wordplay, intending to secure the "acquittal" he was seeking. He did not ask McNaghten whether he intended to kill Sir Robert Peel. Instead, he entered a plea of "not guilty" on the record. At the trial, witnesses to the crime testified that McNaghten appeared to be sane and deliberate in his actions, and acquaintances testified that "he had always seemed perfectly sane."[28] This, however, was a psychiatric show trial. Testifying for the "defense," nine "medical gentlemen"—led by Dr. E. T. Monro, one of the most prominent alienists of the day—unanimously declared that "his [McNaghten's] delusions of persecution meant that 'his moral liberty was destroyed.' The prosecution presented no medical evidence to rebut this."[29]

At the conclusion of the testimony, the solicitor general (the prosecutor) addressed the jury: "Gentlemen of the jury, after the intimation I have received from the Bench I feel that I should not be properly discharging my duties to the Crown and to the public if I asked you to give your verdict in this case *against* the prisoner. . . . This unfortunate man, at the time he committed the act was labouring under insanity; and, of course, if he were so, he would be entitled to his acquittal."[30] I emphasize the word *against* to indicate that the prosecutor considered the decision to imprison McNaghten for life as being *not against* him. McNaghten did not seem disturbed by the prospect of being hanged and did not ask for such "mercy." It was the lawyers and judges who were disturbed by having to order his hanging.

The chief judge, C. J. Tindal, then *instructed the jury to bring in a verdict of not guilty by reason of insanity*:

Tindal, C. J.: If you think you ought to hear the evidence more fully, in that case I will state it to you, and leave the case in your hands. Probably, however, sufficient has now been laid before you, and you will say whether you want further information.

Foreman of the Jury: We require no more, my Lord.

Tindal, C. J.: If you find the prisoner not guilty, say on the ground of insanity, in which case proper care will be taken of him.

Foreman: We find the prisoner not guilty, on the grounds of insanity.[31]

Despite the evidence that McNaghten was "railroaded" from the gallows to the madhouse, historians, scholars, psychiatrists, and lawyers have consistently referred to the McNaghten case as a "trial." But there was no McNaghten *trial*. To call the judicial proceeding against McNaghten a criminal trial is an Orwellian untruth: The prosecution did not proceed *against* McNaghten, it proceeded *for* him. As Judge Tindal put it, "proper *care* will be taken of him." The proper *punishment* for McNaghten would have been death by hanging. *De jure*, McNaghten was treated as if he had been insane when he shot Drummond; *de facto*, he was treated as if he had been, was, and will always remain insane. He was incarcerated in Broadmoor, the first so-called hospital for the criminally insane in England, and died there twenty-one years later.

McNaghten's contemporaries recognized that the jury that sent him to Broadmoor did him no favors. Dr. Forbes Winslow, a leading Victorian alienist, lauded the insanity verdict precisely because it was horrible, not because it was humane:

To talk of a person escaping the extreme penalty of the law on the plea of Insanity, as one being subjected to no kind or degree of *punishment*, is a perfect mockery of truth and perversion of language. Suffer no punishment! He is exposed to the severest pain and torture of body and mind that can be inflicted upon a human creature short of being publicly strangled upon the gallows. If the fact be doubted, let a visit be paid to that dreadful *den* at Bethlehem Hospital . . . where the criminal portion of the establishment are confined like wild beasts in an iron cage![32]

Surveying the fate of insanity acquittees serving life sentences in insane asylums, Roger Smith, the author of a study of Victorian insanity trials, observes: "In practice, a warrant of removal to a criminal asylum usually meant a permanent removal. It was extremely difficult to attribute 'recovery' to someone who had shown potential for violence. . . . Medical superintendents accepted their custodial role."[33] Not much has changed since then.

From Murderous Intent to Homicidal Impulse

Common sense tells us to assume that people kill others and themselves for essentially the same reasons they do anything else; namely, to advance their self-interest as they perceive it. Unable to disprove this assumption, alienists based their arguments on an analogy between certain manifestations of bodily diseases, such as convulsions, and certain alleged manifestations of so-called mental diseases, such as murder. That was the tool Maudsley used to transform the *deliberate intention* of the guilty murderer into the *irresistible impulse* of the innocent madman:

No one now-a-days who is engaged in the treatment of mental disease doubts that he has to do with the disordered function of a bodily organ—of the brain. . . . Disease of mind is a derangement which is nowise metaphysical, but one strictly comparable with such other nervous disorders as neuralgia and convulsions. . . . The question in all such cases [homicidal insanity] obviously is whether the impulse was really irresistible or whether it was only unresisted. . . . That the impulse may be irresistible is beyond question. . . . The truth is, that, what in the sane mind is controllable passion becomes in the insane mind uncontrollable insanity.[34]

Law is based more often on sentiment than reason. This is why, in the case of the insanity excuse, it is not enough to argue that asserting that mental illness causes murder is false. We must also ask, again and again, *Cui bono?*: Who profits from accepting the claim in general and in any particular instance? The answer is: The individuals and institutions that advance it, who, not by coincidence, are the individuals and institutions with their hands on the levers of both the government and the media. Unfortunately, the intellectual timidity even of Maudsley's most distinguished critics, in particular of the Victorian jurist, Sir James Fitzjames Stephen, has rendered the psychiatric perspective on crime and insanity impregnable. Stephen's remarks on the subject, set forth in his magisterial *History of the Criminal Law of England*, merit being quoted at some length:

I have read a variety of medical works on madness, but I have found the greatest difficulty in discovering in any of them the information of which I stood in need. . . . Most of the authors whose works I have read insist at a length which in the present day I should have supposed was unnecessary on the proposition that insanity is a disease, but hardly any of them describe it as a disease is described. They all . . . describe a number of states of mind which do not appear to have any necessary or obvious connection with each other. These they classify . . . these [the mad-doctors'] expressions are like adjectives connected with an unintelligible substantive. To say that a strong and causeless desire to set a house on fire is pyromania . . . is to substitute words for thoughts. It is like telling a man that a whale and a monkey are both mammals, when you do not explain what mammal means. . . . I have sought in vain for what appeared on the face of it to be an accurate picture of "insanity as a real disease" in many medical works.[35]

Instead of inquiring into the practical usefulness of pretending that insanity is a disease, Stephen restated the truism that "all crimes are voluntary actions"[36] and delivered this scathing critique of Maudsley's views:

It is to be recollected in connection with this subject that *though madness is a disease*, it is one which to a great extent and in many cases is the *sufferer's own fault*. In reading medical works the connection between insanity and every sort of repulsive vice is made so clear, that it seems more natural to ask whether in many cases insanity is not rather a crime in itself than an excuse. . . . We do not recognize the grossest ignorance, the most wretched education, the most constant involuntary association with criminals, as an excuse for crime; though in many cases . . . they explain the fact that crimes are committed. This should lead to strictness in admitting insanity as being in doubtful cases any excuse at all for crime, or any reason for mitigating the punishment due to it.[37]

Unable or unwilling to reject the medical model of insanity,* Stephen resorted to attributing insanity to the "sufferer's own fault," a formulation doomed to failure. Still, he stuck to his guns: He insisted that there was no evidence that the insane person is not responsible for his behavior and showed that the methods psychiatrists use to control persons in insane asylums contradict their claims about the nature of insanity: "The principle that madmen ought in some cases to be punished is proved by the practice of lunatic asylums."[38] Stephen recognized that the practice of excusing crime as mental illness "suggests that nobody should ever be punished at all" and that the result is that the authorities entrusted with enforcing the law evade their responsibility and are applauded for doing so: "Reluctance to punish when punishment is needed seems to me not benevolence but cowardice, and I think that the proper attitude of mind toward criminals is not long-suffering charity but open enmity; for the object of the criminal law is to overcome evil with evil."[39]

Stephen's critique of the intellectual weaknesses of the insanity excuse was astute, but he was blind to its political-strategic value. Also, he was excessively respectful of tradition, which probably accounts for his opposition to any relaxation of the laws against suicide. His comment about a proposed revision of the Penal Code that lay before Parliament was: "It

---

*Like many others, Stephen had personal reasons for not asking certain question: both his son and his niece (Virginia Woolf's half-sister) had been committed to mental institutions.

would, I think, be a pity if Parliament were to enact any measure tending to alter the feeling with which it [suicide] is and ought to be regarded."[40]

The Crime of Punishment

By the 1950s, the United States was intoxicated with the ideology of diagnosis-and-treatment as a personal and social panacea. The eighteenth- and nineteenth-century idea of insanity as an excuse was expanded to fill all of human existence: Everyone is, more or less, mentally ill; no one is responsible for his misdeeds. This may sound like a satirical exaggeration. Regrettably, it is not. The following statements are illustrative.

In 1946, with World War II barely concluded, the Canadian psychiatrist G. Brock Chisholm, the highest-ranking medical officer in the Canadian Armed Forces during World War II, declared: "The reinterpretation and eventual eradication of the concepts of right and wrong . . . are the belated objectives of practically all effective psychotherapy. . . . If the race is to be freed of its crippling burden of good and evil it must be psychiatrists who take the original responsibility."[41]

In 1963, Karl Menninger (1893–1990) published his hugely popular book, *The Vital Balance*. In it, he wrote: "We say that all people have mental illnesses of different degrees at different times . . . and this is precisely what recent epidemiological studies have demonstrated. . . . Gone forever is the notion that the mentally ill person is an exception. It is now accepted that most people have some degree of mental illness at some time."[42] In his book *The Crime of Punishment*, published in 1968, Menninger maintained that *all* criminals are mentally ill and ought to be treated, not punished. To be sure, "Some mental patients must be detained for a time even against their wishes."[43]

The idea of excusing the self-killer by attributing to him the fictitious malady called "insanity" was invented as a tactic for the merciful treatment of his survivors. It was too good a gambit to be limited to a suicide. In the United States today, there is virtually no situation in which the notion of mental illness may not be brought into play to diminish or annul the actor's responsibility for his action; to deny his role as moral agent and redefine him as a victim; and to hold others responsible for the deleterious consequences of his behavior. By the same token, virtually no behavior deemed undesirable by authorities is immune from being subjected to "therapeutic" social controls.

The more society relies on therapeutic controls, the more their use reinforces belief in the reality of mental illness and, generally, in the rationale of treating bad habits as if they were diseases. In the process, the public loses sight of the fact that bad habits are not diseases; that diagnosing (mis)behaviors does not make them diseases; and that psychiatrists have nothing to do with treating diseases, but have everything to do with regulating behavior.

The insanity defense is not merciful. Involuntary mental hospitalization is not a treatment. Both are coercive methods of social control. Both rest on attributing an absence of *mens rea* to the actor. Both result in the "protected" person's being deprived of liberty. Both function as tactical weapons in psychiatry's war on dignity, liberty, and responsibility.

4

"Preventing" Suicide

"Saving" Lives

People are being forced to continue to live a life that has become unbearable for them for valid reasons. . . . Even if a few more [patients] killed themselves, does this reason justify the fact that we torture hundreds of patients and aggravate their disease?

—Eugen Bleuler (1857–1939)[1]

We give ECT [electroconvulsive therapy] to such a [suicidal] patient . . . daily until mental confusion supervenes and reduces the ability of the patient to carry out his suicidal drive.

—American Handbook of Psychiatry (1974)[2]

Never kill yourself while you are suicidal.

—Edwin Shneidman (1996)[3]

The words *preventing* and *saving* in the chapter title are placed between quotation marks to indicate that both terms function here as euphemisms. The term "preventing" conceals the indignity and injuriousness of psychiatric coercion. The term "saving" implies that suicide prevention programs save lives. Since suicide prevention (SP) rests on the use of coercive psychiatric practices, it ought to be called "coercive psychiatric suicide prevention" (CPSP).

"The public health significance of death by suicide," declares an editorial in the *American Journal of Public Health*, "has been emphasized by the recent establishment of the National Center for Injury Prevention and Control at the Center for Disease Control. The principal goal of the new Center is the identification of effective suicide prevention methods."[4]

The die is now cast. Disapproved behaviors of all sorts are defined as diseases, and approved behaviors of all sorts are defined as treatments. The concepts of *disease* and *treatment* are now thoroughly politicized. Doctors, judges, journalists, civil libertarians, everyone accepts, or pretends to accept, that killing oneself without physician approval is a disease justifying State coercion, and that killing oneself with physician approval is a treatment justifying State exemption from the strictures of drug prohibition. Not surprisingly, these novel concepts of disease and treatment conflict with the traditional meaning of "helping" as aiding a person to attain his self-chosen goal or persuading him to change it. Helping a person against his will—that is, forcing him to pursue a goal he does not want to pursue—is a contradiction of terms. Joining suicide prevention and coercion as if they were indissolubly united makes us neglect the possibilities of noncoercive suicide prevention, an option we cannot consider so long as we view suicide as the consequence of untreated (mental-brain) disease.

Suicide prevention is a modern idea, the product of the concept of suicide as a sickness and its prevention as a species of disease prevention. It is a counterproductive policy that rests on a fallacious analogy: Suicide may be said to be *like* a disease, but it is not a disease. Some years ago I proposed comparing the would-be suicide with the would-be emigrant: One wants to leave life, the other wants to leave his homeland.[5] Killing oneself is a decision, not a disease. The political analogy fits it more closely than does the medical analogy.*

One of the most important differences between free and totalitarian countries is that people can leave the former without permission by authorities of the State, but they can leave the latter only with their explicit authorization. The coercive psychiatric prevention of suicide resembles the coercive political prevention of emigration: Psychiatric bureaucrats insist that the would-be suicide should not leave his life, much as totalitarian bureaucrats insist that the would-be emigrant must not leave his country. The sincerity or cynicism of the agents does not matter; what matters is the coerced person's loss of liberty, justified by patriotic or psychiatric rationalization and rhetoric. To one who believes in benevolent coercion, the beneficiary who rejects his benefactor and wants to vote with his feet perforce appears to be bad or mad or both, and must therefore be forcibly prevented from doing what he wants to do. "What's a government for," asks National Public Radio correspondent Susan Stamberg, "if it doesn't step in and say, 'You can't commit suicide'?"[6]

PUNISHMENT MASQUERADING AS TREATMENT

If a person fears that he might kill himself and seeks help because he considers *that* a problem, we do not say that he is receiving a "suicide preven-

*I did not realize then that Thomas Jefferson had used the same analogy. See the Appendix.

tion service." We call such a service "psychotherapy." Trying to persuade another person to refrain from an action which we believe is injurious to his best medical, moral, or financial interests is always permissible and may or may not be meritorious; however, that does not justify replacing suasion with coercion. We reserve the term "suicide prevention" for interventions such as the following:

- A young man fails to return home. His relatives call the police and say they fear he may be suicidal. The police find the man in the woods and *arrest him "on a charge of violation of the Mental Health Law."*[7]

- A man calls the Los Angeles Suicide Prevention Center and says he wants to shoot himself. When the worker asks for his address, he refuses to give it. "Silently but urgently, [the worker] signaled a co-worker to begin *tracing the call.* . . . An agonizing 40 minutes passed. Then she heard the voice of a policeman come on the phone to say the man was safe."[8]

- A man threatens to jump from an overpass to the highway below. Police officers arrive: " 'We told him we wouldn't hurt him and just wanted to help.' . . . When he climbed back over, the officers ran to him and *handcuffed him.*" The man was taken to a mental hospital.[9]

If a person is determined to kill himself and is physically able to do so, it is virtually impossible to prevent his suicide. This truism is regularly documented by newspaper stories. In March 1997, Pittsburgh police discovered the dismembered body of a woman in the basement of a condemned row house. The tenement's owner was arrested by the police and placed in the back of the police van. The man was "shackled and his hands were cuffed behind his back in the van, yet he still managed to remove his belt, loop it around the grating, and hang himself during the 12-minute ride to the police station."[10]

The Semantics of Suicide Prevention

The practice of SP rests on civil commitment, that is, the involuntary detention of the subject in a building called "hospital." Is such a place of detention a hospital or a prison? *Webster's Dictionary* defines prison as: "A place or condition of confinement or restraint." *Black's Law Dictionary* offers the following definitions: "[Prevent, v.] To hinder, frustrate, prohibit, impede, or preclude; to obstruct; to intercept. . . . [Prison] A public building or other place for the confinement or safe custody of persons, whether as a punishment imposed by the law or otherwise in the course of the administration of justice."[11]

Linking the terms "suicide" and "prevention" is an abuse of language, similar to linking the terms "mental" and "hospital." "Prevention" and "hospital" imply consent and cooperation. Only when a woman wants to avert her own pregnancy do we speak of "preventing pregnancy." When the State uses force to prevent a woman who wants to become pregnant from becoming pregnant, we call the intervention "forcible sterilization." By the same token, when a psychiatrist uses the power of the State to prevent a person who wants to kill himself from killing himself, we should call the intervention "coercive psychiatric suicide prevention" and we should regard it as a punishment, not as a treatment. Regardless of the coercer's intention, the person whose freedom is abridged experiences the abridgment as punishment. When a mother tells her son to go to his room and stay there for an hour, he perceives it as punishment. To say that her intention is to correct the child's behavior does not invalidate his experiencing her action as punishment, nor does it negate the likelihood that her intention may be punitive as well. As long as we pretend that procedures called "treatments" *ipso facto* help the recipients, and procedures called "punishments" *ipso facto* harm them, we foreclose the possibility of an open-minded examination of these interventions.

Individuals, groups, and the State regularly use actual or threatened punishment to prevent, or try to prevent, people from engaging in certain behaviors, for example, selling and buying certain books or drugs. In every such situation the persons prevented from realizing their intentions regard the restraint as a form of *unjust and unmerited punishment*. It is disingenuous to expect that the person forcibly restrained in the name of suicide prevention should regard his situation differently. Indeed, the cruelty of his punishment is compounded by the fact that his physician and his family insist that they are helping him, thus invalidating his perception that they are harming him.

FROM EXCUSING SELF-MURDER TO PREVENTING SUICIDE

When the person who killed himself was regarded as a self-murderer, the penalties the Law inflicted on his corpse and family were thought of as measures intended to prevent suicide, just as we think of imprisoning drug dealers and executing murderers as measures intended to prevent drug abuse and murder.

However, once the self-murderer was transformed from a criminal-victimizer into a patient-victim, punishment could no longer be viewed or used as a preventive measure. Only bad people or bad deeds deserve "punishment." Sick people and disease deserve "treatment." Defining the suicide as sick ("insane") set the stage for preventing and treating suicide *as if* it were a disease and marks the birth of modern psychiatry:

1. The attribution of suicide to (the fiction of) mental illness is emblematic of psychiatric theory.
2. The posthumous defense of the successful self-killer as a patient not responsible for his (prohibited) act is emblematic of the social function of psychiatry.
3. The use of coercion as suicide prevention (involuntary mental hospitalization) is emblematic of psychiatric practice.

Linking suicide to mental illness and mental illness to irrationality has serious consequences, some probably unintended. For example, if an intellectually creative person kills himself, the value of his cognitive productions is likely to be undermined and even destroyed. In contrast, probably because art and madness are supposed to partake of the same mystery, the suicide of an artist is likely to enhance his work. The suicides of Otto Weininger and Bruno Bettelheim, on the one hand, and of Vincent van Gogh and Sylvia Plath, on the other, are illustrative. These facts make so-called suicide education an exercise in hypocrisy, as the following story illustrates.

In 1994, Jonah Eskin hanged himself after finishing his freshman year at the West Orange [NJ] High School.[12] An excellent student, Eskin was especially gifted in music. However, his school yearbook omitted his picture and the school board rejected his mother's effort to establish a music scholarship in his name. When she persisted, she discovered that the school board had a policy "which had prohibited any memorial for a student or staff member who committed suicide, . . . [lest it] would tend to glorify the death and possibly lead to copycat cases." The school principal told Mrs. Eskin: "If I allow you to do this, some poor, desperate, lonely soul will do this just to get a scholarship in his name."

Suicide experts support this policy. Dr. Alan Berman, the executive director of the American Association of Suicidology, stated: "They [students] see a tribute and think, I, too, will be appreciated after my death." Dr. Michael Peck, an expert on youth suicide, agreed: "Schools needs to be extremely careful how they proceed with any memorial, for fear of copycat suicides." The students are not fooled. "I don't know for whose good they were doing this," remarked a 17-year-old boy at Jonah Eskin's school. "By trying to bury his memory, they brought much more attention to his death than it would have gotten in the first place."

Justifying the Uses of Psychiatric Power

The practice of medicine began as a consensual relationship: The sick person, seeking relief from *his* suffering, assumed the patient role voluntarily. By contrast, the practice of psychiatry began as a coercive relationship: The alienist, enlisted by the troublesome person's relatives seeking relief from *their* suffering, imposed the patient role on the subject against his will.

The medicalization of madness and the (quasi-)criminalization of the madman were needed, and continue to be needed, to reconcile man's quixotic quest for maximizing his liberty and minimizing his responsibility; the former animated the Rule of Law, the latter the Rule of Mental Health. The Rule of Law means equality before the law and a system of government constrained by law. The Rule of Mental Health means individualized justice as "treatment" and a system of government unconstrained by law—that is, by considerations of the subject's innocence or guilt. In other words, the Rule of Mental Health enshrines the principle of *parens patriae* (the State as parent) not only toward minors but also toward adults successfully incriminated as "dangerous to themselves or others." In effect, the rule is: liberty for the mentally healthy Self; psychiatry for the mentally ill Other. Not surprisingly, the idea of insanity—as an illness that justifies incarcerating the patient in his own best interest—was invented by those who wanted him incarcerated, namely, members of the dominant classes of seventeenth-century English society.

Medieval English guardianship procedures for "idiots" lent support to the emerging practice of mad-housing "lunatics." Both interventions grew out of, and implemented, the feudal tradition of preserving landed wealth and ensuring its stable transfer in the family. The procedures for declaring a person incompetent and a lunatic were similar: "Commissions examined such persons before a jury that ruled on their sanity. . . . *Physicians played essentially no role in the certification process itself.*"[13] Long before pauper lunatics were imprisoned in insane asylums, propertied persons declared mad were deprived of liberty in a style befitting their station: "Physical supervision and care of the disabled party was commonly handled by retaining a live-in servant, the so-called 'lunatic's keeper,' a person usually of the same gender as the disabled individual. . . . Boarding out the lunatic or idiot at a private dwelling, in the company of a servant, was also commonplace."[14*]

Except for historians of psychiatry, few people realize that the early madhouses were not hospitals. They were the keepers' private homes, into which they took a few men and women, often only one or two, as *involuntary* boarders or houseguests. The individuals who owned and operated these "private homes" were mainly clergymen. There was sound historical and legal reason for this: The practice of healing began as an undifferentiated religious-medical enterprise. When the social world split into sacred and profane parts, the practice of healing also split: one part became religious and spiritual, the other part, secular and materialist.

---

*From the thirteenth century on, English common law recognized two classes of incompetents: idiots, mentally subnormal from birth, considered permanently impaired; and lunatics, normal persons who went mad, considered capable of recovery.

Western tradition sanctions interpreting insanity in religious terms, attributing it to demonic possession, treating it by means of exorcism, and accepting clerical coercion as morally laudable and legitimate. When people believed that eternal life in the hereafter was more important than a brief sojourn on earth, exorcizing the possessed person by torturing him, to improve the quality of his life after death, was perceived as an act of beneficence. A long history of lawful coercion in the name of salvation testified to and justified the priest's use of therapeutic force.

The Galenic physicians' refusal to control (mis)behavior as malady was consistent with their historical role of treating only voluntary patients. The priests' role was altogether different: They had long served the interests of both rulers and ruled, which accounts for their role as trailblazing experts on madness and as pioneer madhouse keepers. Thus, when Englishmen first tried to use doctors to dispose of their problematic relatives, the physicians declined the invitation, a scenario illustrated by Macbeth's encounter with the doctor he summons, ostensibly to cure his wife.

As the prestige of Science replaced that of Religion, psychiatric coercion replaced theological coercion. The alienist's alliance with the State and the popular legitimation of his power soon led to the acceptance of mad-housing as the proper social method for controlling troublesome persons. *Pari passu*, the practice of medicalized coercion—unconstrained by the safeguards of the English criminal justice system, yet intrinsic to the operation of the madhouse business—generated recurrent protests against the so-called abuses of mad-doctoring. The principle of nonrestraint and the so-called moral treatment of insanity are best regarded in this light—that is, as manifestations of the mad-doctors' dissatisfaction with their role as coercers. Not surprisingly, this uneasiness could not be remedied by cosmetic reforms: The ideal of nonrestraint was incompatible with the reality of the mad-doctor's mandate to prevent suicide.

In 1796, the Quaker philanthropist William Tuke founded the York Retreat, which, under the management of his grandson, Samuel Tuke (1784–1857), became a celebrated institution. (Neither Tuke was a physician.) Samuel Tuke offered this optimistic account of the practice of nonrestraint:

Neither chains nor corporal punishments are tolerated, on any pretext, in this establishment. . . . To the mild system of treatment adopted at the Retreat, I have no doubt we may partly attribute the happy recovery of so large a proportion of melancholy patients. . . . If it be true, that oppression makes a wise man mad, is it to be supposed that stripes, and insults, and injuries, for which the receiver knows no cause, are calculated to make a madman wise? Or would they not exasperate his disease, and excite his resentment?[15]

How did the practitioners of nonrestraint reconcile their avowed principles with their presumed duty to protect the mad person from killing himself? They didn't. Tuke himself acknowledged that "Coercion, when requisite, is considered as a necessary evil."[16] Alas, the principle of nonrestraint, celebrated in books on the history of psychiatry, never existed in practice.[17] Noncoercive mad-doctoring was, and noncoercive psychiatry remains, an oxymoron.[18]

Suicide Prevention and the Social Role of the Psychiatrist

Regardless of what we call it, legally sanctioned coercive detention to prevent harm, to self or others, is *preventive detention*. Part of the appeal of the Therapeutic State lies in letting us simultaneously reject preventive detention as a legal-judicial abuse and embrace it as beneficial prevention-and-treatment of mental illness. Despite the impossibility of preventing suicide and the legal risks entailed in promising to prevent it, virtually all psychiatrists consider it their professional duty to prevent suicide, typically asserting: "Of all professional groups, psychiatrists have the most important part to play in suicide prevention."[19]

The psychiatric argument for SP may be summarized as follows: Suicide is the result of mental illness; mental illness is a treatable disorder; adequate treatment of mental illness eliminates the cause of suicide and prevents the fatal outcome; *ergo*, suicide prevention is a life-saving medical treatment. Edwin Shneidman, the father of American suicidology, puts it this way: "Suicide prevention is like fire prevention."[20] In other words, Shneidman sees suicide as unintentional, similar to a forest fire caused by lightning: Action is like oxidation, the prevention of *willed human behavior* is like the prevention of the *combustion of a material object*. The foundation on which the vast structure of CPSP rests may be weak, but the fear of suicide is strong. As a result, every effort to prevent suicide, regardless of the means employed, appears to be meritorious, while every abstention from such an effort, regardless of the principles it serves to uphold, appears to be an act of "medical negligence" or worse. There are more than two hundred organizations in the United States concerned with suicide prevention and not a single organization opposing the practice.[21]

The belief that suicide is due to mental illness forms the keystone in the arch that supports not only CPSP but psychiatry itself. The stone is small, but the arch it caps is strong enough to uphold a massive structure. The intellectual foundation of psychiatry may be insubstantial, its moral foundations rotten, and its scientific foundation nonexistent, but the fear of suicide alone is powerful enough to preclude reasoned debate about CPSP, much less deviation from its practice.

Modern writers on SP fall into two classes. The majority regard self-killing as a disease similar to contagious diseases, injurious to both self and others; they support suicide prevention as analogous to the prevention of communicable diseases. A minority regard suicide as a nondisease, yet, they, too, advocate preventing and treating it as if it were a disease and support suicide prevention as the thwarting of "unreasonable, self-destructive behavior."

Edwin S. Shneidman's writings exemplify the majority view. His rhetoric—sprinkled liberally with phrases such as "clinical core," "case histories," and "psychological autopsy"—exposes his premises and the conclusions they entail.[22] He declares: "Stripped down to its bones, my argument goes like this: in almost every case, suicide is caused by pain, a certain kind of pain—*psychological* pain, which I call *psychache.* . . . [Suicide] is a lonely act, a desperate, and almost always, *unnecessary* one."[23] There are exceptions, however; for example, Nazi Field Marshall Erwin Rommel's suicide, which Shneidman says was ordered by Hitler: "The onus here is on the *demented* Hitler."[24] Pursuing the image of a demented dictator as a suicide pathogen, Shneidman adds: "Every single instance of suicide is an action by the dictator or emperor of your mind. But in every case of suicide, the person is getting bad advice from a part of that mind, the inner chamber of councilors, who are temporarily in a panicked state and in no position to serve the person's best long-range interests."[25] His conclusion: "Never kill yourself while you are suicidal."[26] *Mutatis mutandis*: "Never eat while you are hungry," "Never have sex while you are aroused," and so forth.

Robert W. Firestone's writings exemplify the minority view. He rejects the claim that suicide is due to mental illness: "I support the view that mental illness is an illusion or myth." Nevertheless he advocates preventing and treating suicide as the thwarting of "unreasonable, self-destructive behavior"[27] and by what he views as "the *obvious fact* that in suicide, *the basic rights of other human beings are being violated.* . . . It is almost impossible for an individual not to be psychologically impaired by a loved one's suicide. . . . The suicide of a loved one, especially a parent, seriously damages the psyches of the survivors, which leads to a social pressure to harm oneself."[28] This claim is patently false: The suicide of a loved one does not always damage the psyches of the survivors. And even if it were true, that would justify only the moral condemnation of suicide, not its forcible prevention. There is no reason to believe that Socrates's disciples were damaged by the suicide of their master. Nor is there reason to believe that the psyche of a 60-year-old man is necessarily damaged by the suicide of his disabled 85-year-old parent. On the contrary, suicide may be experienced as a liberation by both the subject and his survivors. Admittedly, the effect of the parent's suicide on his minor child is a more complicated matter. However, we cannot know whether the parent, had he remained alive, would have been a beneficial or harmful influence on his child's life; and therefore, any generalization about the effect of parental suicide on children must be false.

Any major event in a person's life—emigration, illness, marriage, divorce, the death of a parent or spouse—may impair or improve a person's ability to cope with life, may hinder or hone his skills, or may dull or deepen his sensitivity to the plight of his fellow man. The result depends partly on the nature of other people's influence on the subject, and largely on the decisions he makes that we call his "adaptation" to the event.

Does "Suicide Prevention" Prevent Suicide?

The answer to that question is a flat-out no. Not only is there absolutely no evidence that CPSP reduces the frequency of suicide; what evidence there is suggests that the practice is likely to increase it. The late Jonas Robitscher cogently observed: "Free mental health services, particularly when other meaningful forms of help are absent, are seductive. . . . Cities where suicide prevention services are offered, for example, show a rise and not a fall in suicides . . . there is the possibility—not sufficiently studied—that the services do actually engender pathology."[29]

A group of investigators reviewed published studies and "concluded that the suicide prevention center does not reach the highest risk population and it may possibly shape the low-risk person toward the act."[30] A report published in a January 1998 issue of *Psychiatric News*, the American Psychiatric Association's official newspaper, informed the reader that "despite decades of progress in developing psychiatric medications, there has been little change in the rate of suicide in the last quarter century."[31] Even Erwin Stengel, one of the most respected advocates of SP, acknowledged that instead of reducing the incidence of suicide, "the triumphs of scientific medicine [have], on the contrary, tended to increase it."[32]

However, SP programs are counterproductive not because of the "triumphs of scientific medicine," but because of the *threats and terrors of psychiatric incarceration*, on which they depend. Ernest Hemingway, Sylvia Plath, and Virginia Woolf are only a few of the famous persons whose suicides may, in part at least, have been provoked by the fear of psychiatric incarceration and involuntary psychiatric treatment. The necessity to make this point is evidence of the biased character of the professional literature on suicide and of the media's uncritical acceptance of the benevolence of psychiatric coercion. Antonin Artaud knew better. He wrote: "I myself spent nine years in an insane asylum and I never had the obsession of suicide, but I know that each conversation with a psychiatrist, every morning at the time of his visit, made me want to hang myself, realizing that I would not be able to slit his throat."[33]

Without fully acknowledging the central role that coercion plays in rendering SP counterproductive, L. D. Hankoff and Bernice Einsidler note that the only SP program "associated with a reduction in the suicide rate . . . [is] the telephone service operated by the Samaritans in England. . . . The Samaritans emphasize that their activities are devoid of all coercive potential . . . even in the face of obvious suicidal plan on the part of the client. The suicidal individual is aware that there will be no interference with his freedom as a result of his contact with the Samaritans."[34]

Nevertheless, most (American) psychiatrists resolutely defend CPSP. It is psychiatric doctrine that the psychiatrist has a professional duty to "protect the patient from his own [suicidal] wishes."[35] This creed follows inexorably from the psychiatrist's perception of the suicidal person as a kind of existential Siamese twin, one wanting to die, the other to live. The psychiatrist diagnoses the suicidal twin as irrational and ill, and the nonsuicidal twin as rational and healthy; he concludes that both need his help, the former to protect him from his illness, the latter, to protect him from his (self)murderous twin. He proceeds to incarcerate the patient in a mental hospital. Intoxicated with the cause of suicide prevention, the psychiatrist inverts Patrick Henry's "Give *me* liberty, or give me death!" declaring: "Give *him (the patient)* commitment, give him drugs, give him electric shock treatment, give him lobotomy, but do not let him choose death!" By so radically illegitimizing another person's wish to die, the suicide-preventer redefines the aspiration of the Other as not an aspiration at all. The result is the utter infantilization and dehumanization of the suicidal person.

Interestingly, political philosophers have long recognized and rejected the *political version* of this line of reasoning as specious and self-serving, but they have refused to confront or confute its *psychiatric version*. Isaiah Berlin's refutation of this form of therapeutic tyranny is not original but it is well stated. He wrote:

The notion of positive freedom has led, historically, to even more frightful perversions. Who orders my life? I do. I? Ignorant, confused, driven hither and thither by uncontrollable passions and drives. . . . Is there not within me a higher, more rational, freer self, able to understand and dominate passions, ignorance, and other defects, which I can attain to only by a process of education or understanding, a process which can be managed only by those who are wiser than myself, who make me aware of my true, "real," deepest self, of what I am at my best? This is a well-known metaphysical view . . . since I am not perhaps sufficiently rational myself, I must obey those who are indeed rational, and who therefore know what is best not only for themselves but also for me. . . . I may feel hemmed in—indeed, crushed—by these authorities, but that is an illusion: when I have grown up and have attained to a fully mature, "real" self, I shall understand that I would have done for me if I had been wise, when I was in an inferior condition, as they are now. . . . There is no despot in the world who cannot use this method of argument for the vilest oppression, in the name of an ideal self which he is seeking to bring to fruition by his own, perhaps somewhat brutal and *prima facie* morally odious means (*prima facie* only for the lower empirical self). The "engineer of human souls," to use Stalin's phrase, knows best . . . whether the tyranny issues from a Marxist leader, a king, a fascist dictator, the masters of an authoritarian Church or class or State, it seeks for the imprisoned "real" self within men, and "liberates" it, so that this self can attain to the level of those who give the orders.[36]

In the absence of a similar political-philosophical critique of the Therapeutic State by respected authorities in political philosophy, the media and the public accept that mental illness is an illness like, say, appendicitis. A patient dying as a result of unprevented suicide is like a patient dying of an inflamed appendix negligently allowed to rupture, and it is therefore the psychiatrist's duty to prevent suicide, by force if necessary. It does not matter that mental illness is unlike appendicitis; that voluntary death by suicide is unlike involuntary death from a ruptured appendix; and that if the two conditions were in fact similar, the psychiatrist could not treat the so-called patient without his consent. The claim that "mental illness is like any other illness," especially when it is advanced in the context of SP, does not provide empirical evidence for it or logical reasoning for why we should believe it. Instead, its purpose is to provide moral and rhetorical justification for an established social practice.

A critical look at legal rulings shows that SP has nothing to do with medicine or treatment, but has everything to do with "custody and control." The parents of a young man who committed suicide while receiving pastoral counseling sued for damages. The court dismissed the plaintiff's claim, stating: "One is ordinarily not liable for actions of another and is under no duty to protect another from harm, *absent special relationship of custody or control.*"[37] (I shall say more about this case presently.) Psychiatrists are held legally liable for the harms their patients inflict on themselves largely because they claim that they have a duty to exercise custody and control over them.

Trying to prevent a person from killing himself is not a sophisticated professional performance that rests on recondite knowledge or skills. Just as preventing anyone from doing anything he wants to do, carrying out such a task requires granting the preventer virtually unlimited power over the subject; depriving the subject of the means and opportunity to kill himself; and keeping the subject in that condition until it is "safe" to set him at liberty without risking that he will kill himself. In practice, this is obviously impossible. Because it is impossible, psychiatrists enjoy (if that is the right word) virtually unlimited professional discretion to employ the most destructive suicide-prevention measures imaginable, provided the measures are called "treatments." The authoritative *American Handbook of Psychiatry*

(1959 edition) endorsed lobotomy "for patients who are threatened with disability or suicide and for whom no other method seems likely to relieve or restore them."[38] In the 1974 edition, lobotomy was replaced by electro-shock treatment administered in sufficient doses to destroy the subject's will to kill himself: "[W]e do advocate its initial use for one type of patient, the agitated patient, often middle-aged and usually a man, who presents frank suicidal intention. We give ECT [electroconvulsive therapy] to such a patient . . . daily until mental confusion supervenes and reduces the ability of the patient to carry out his suicidal drive."[39]

The lay person who hears the term "suicide prevention" is unlikely to suspect that psychiatrists have the power, and are heartless enough, to impose such measures on individuals in the name of preventing suicide.

SUICIDE AS A PUBLIC HEALTH PROBLEM

Webster's Dictionary defines the term "public health" as "The art and science dealing with the protection and improvement of community health by organized community effort." Traditionally, the term denoted activities undertaken by a governmental agency, using the economic and coercive powers of the State, to protect groups (the inhabitants of a city, military personnel) from disease-causing agents or conditions in the environment. Typical public health measures are sanitation (sewage disposal, the provision of clean water and pure food) and the control of infectious diseases (protection from microbial diseases, such as cholera and typhoid). By contrast, measures that individuals can take to protect themselves from disease or injury have traditionally been viewed as matters of *private health* (a term I use here to underscore the distinction between it and public health).

Private Behavior as Public Health Problem

Today's State controls of personal behavior, justified by appeals to physical and mental health, closely resemble yesterday's State controls of personal behavior, justified by appeals to spiritual health. Thomas Jefferson recognized this problem at a very early stage. In the birth year of the United States, he issued this warning: "The care of every man's soul belongs to himself. But what if he neglects the care of it? Well what if he neglects the care of his health or estate, which more nearly relates to the state. Will the magistrate make a law that he shall not be poor or sick? Laws provide against injury from others; but not from ourselves. God himself will not save men against their wills."[40]

Interventions justified in the name of health—defined as therapeutic not punitive—fall outside the scope of the criminal law and are therefore exempt from constitutional restraints on state coercion. Promoted as protecting the best interests of both the patients *and* the public, such measures are viewed as valuable public services. Therein, precisely, lies the danger.

Freedom means the opportunity to act wisely or unwisely, to help or harm ourselves. Free access to a particular drug, like free access to any object, increases our opportunities for both using and abusing it. Because it is true that no man is an island, and because every private act may be deemed to harm not only the actor's best interests, but also the economic, existential, medical, or religious well-being of others, no private behavior is safe from being classified as a public health problem and from being controlled by means of medical sanctions.

What is private and what is not—where we draw the line between the private sphere and the public sphere or whether we draw such a line at all—is a matter of convention. Ever since the beginning of this century, especially in recent decades, we have been moving toward redefining certain personal choices as public health problems. The 1997 Washington State "Drug Medicalization and Prevention Act" is an example. The act asserts that "we need to . . . recognize that drug abuse and addiction are public health problems that should be treated as diseases."[41] This interpretation flies in the face of the common-sense secular view that what we put into our bodies is a matter of *private health, not public health.* If the State lets us poison ourselves slowly with cigarettes, by what logic or right can it prevent us from poisoning ourselves quickly with barbiturates? In the privacy of their minds, many people might still acknowledge that killing oneself is, or ought to be, recognized as a private (family) affair.

Suicide: Escaping the Trap

The motives for suicide are no more abnormal or arcane than are the motives for other acts. People kill themselves because they find life so unpleasant—so mentally or physically painful, so humiliating and hopeless—that dying seems to them more attractive than living. Biographers, novelists, playwrights, and poets have given us eloquent descriptions of the inner and outer circumstances of people who chose to die by suicide. As an abstract generalization we may say that the suicide is a person who *feels trapped, often because he has suffered a grave defeat.* The defeats that most damage a person's will to live are loss of child, spouse, or lover; loss of health, especially mobility; loss of income or savings; and loss of honor, reputation, or status. The individual so trapped may decide that the best way out of this is through the door marked "death."

It follows that if we want to avoid killing ourselves, we must try to avoid becoming trapped. Living a virtuous life may be regarded as an effective program of personal suicide prevention: Frugality forestalls want; useful labor averts anomie; honesty protects against scandal. It also follows that it is impossible to protect others from becoming trapped. The mere effort is incompatible with this and every other culture: Religion, Law, a free press, informal social sanctions, all entail potential punishments and hence entrapments. Many people live lives of crime, deceit, and imposture. Some are exposed, feel trapped, and kill themselves. Here are two dramatic examples.

- On May 16, 1996, about to be unmasked by *Newsweek* for wearing two medals that he was never awarded, Jeremy Boorda—the first Jewish enlisted man to rise to the rank of Admiral in the U.S. Navy—shot himself through the heart.[42]
- On May 31, 1996, Nicholas L. Bissell Jr.—chief prosecutor for Somerset County, NJ, from 1982 until his death in 1996—was "convicted on 30 counts of mail fraud, income-tax evasion, embezzlement, abuse of power, and failure of his sworn duty to uphold the law." After a 13-year reign of terror, during which he specialized in "luring drug suspects with valuable assets into Somerset County so the prosecutor's office could seize their property," Bissell was indicted, convicted, and released on bail, wearing an electronic bracelet, and awaiting a 10-year prison sentence. He fled to Nevada and shot himself to death in a motel.[43]

Accounts of less sensational suicides provoked by the subject's legal predicament, such as the following, are frequently reported in the newspapers:

- "A Purdue University freshman facing drug charges fatally shot the dorm counselor who reported him to the police, then locked himself in his bedroom and killed himself."[44]
- "A Fullerton, California man facing a misdemeanor charge killed himself because he mistakenly believed he faced a lengthy 'three-strikes' prison term. Clinton J. Warner, 22, shot himself in the head. . . . He left behind a note saying he was worried about going to prison for life."[45]

These men not only broke the law; they were also caught doing so. Had they not been caught, they might still be alive. Did catching them *cause* their suicide? This may sound like a satirical question, but it is not. It has become so politically incorrect to attribute suicide to the subject's decision to kill himself that it is culturally more plausible to hold persons other than the suicide responsible for the act than it is to hold the subject himself responsible for it. Sometimes people blame the press for "hounding the victim" to his death. Sometimes the press blames parents and the State for failing to recognize the mental illness of a killer or self-killer and thus fail to prevent murder and suicide. In November 1997, *The New Yorker* published a feature story on the life and death of John C. Salvi III. The caption read: "A year after John Salvi's suicide in prison, questions are being raised about why . . . his parents and the state didn't recognize his mental illness when they saw it."[46] *A priori,* the author of the article rejects the interpretation that Salvi might have killed his victims because of his moral convictions and himself because he felt guilty for what he had done.

Salvi pleaded insanity, was convicted of murder, and was sentenced to life imprisonment. Eight months later, he killed himself by tying a plastic garbage can liner around his neck. James L. Sultan, the attorney appointed by the court to work on Salvi's appeal, declared: "He belonged in a hospital." Salvi's mother complained "that she had been telling people for a long time and no one wanted to listen that her son suffered from 'long term mental illness.' "[47] In January 1997, the Commonwealth of Massachusetts set aside his conviction: "To John and Anne-Marie [Salvi], at least, the ruling meant that their son was absolved of his crimes—'innocent by reason of insanity,' his mother says."[48]

Coercive Psychiatric Suicide Prevention: The *Furor Therapeuticus* of Our Age

Notwithstanding the history of the twentieth century, one enthusiast for CPSP goes so far as to assert that "even if a person does not value his own life, Western society does value everyone's life. . . . No one in contemporary Western society would suggest that people be allowed to commit suicide as they please without some attempt to intervene or prevent such suicides."[49]* The premise is false and the conclusion is a *non sequitur.* The Christian martyr wanted to end his life *precisely because he valued it in principle,* but valued it no longer in the existential state in which he found himself. Similarly, the suicidal person today is likely to want to end his life although he too values it, but not in the existential state in which he finds himself.

The claim that Western society values the patient's life more highly than does the patient himself is rubbish. The patient is a complete stranger to the psychiatrist. Why should he value the patient's life more highly than does the patient himself? This claim is also inconsistent with the psychiatrist's insistence that he is a doctor like any other. The family physician does not assert that he values his diabetic patient's life more highly than does the patient who fails to take his insulin. Although the medical patient suffers from a real (bodily) disease, which is often readily controlled by simple and safe therapeutic procedures, the law recognizes the patient's right to reject treatment. In contrast, the mental patient, who suffers from no demonstrable disease and whose desire to commit suicide has regularly been shown to be

---

*Note the similarity between this language and the language of religious intolerance: "No one would suggest that people be allowed to deny the divinity of Jesus, mock Mohammed, and so on."

unresponsive to psychiatric intervention, is deprived of the right to reject treatment.

Diagnosing and treating diabetes and glaucoma prevent hyperglycemic coma and blindness far more effectively than diagnosing and treating depression prevent suicide. Nevertheless, nonpsychiatric physicians do not seek the privilege to impose their diagnoses and treatments on patients against their will, perhaps because they know that they can always count on psychiatrists as repositories for their unwanted patients. That is why psychiatrists are useful for physicians. Psychiatrists know this and, to maintain their usefulness, they cling to the power to treat patients against their will.

The modern psychiatrist insists that mental illnesses are "treatable" and that, if the patient rejects treatment, psychiatric intervention ought to be imposed on him by force. This is a pathognomonic sign of *furor therapeuticus*, an ailment most likely to affect physicians when they are most helpless.* In the past, this *furor* led to bloodletting as a panacea, with George Washington as one of its most distinguished victims. Today, it leads to the use of so-called psychiatric drugs as a panacea for mental diseases, especially for "patients" who refuse to assume the patient role: The most conspicuous victims of contemporary *furor therapeuticus* are children and old persons. There is bitter irony in this situation. When the physician has an effective treatment for a real disease, he and the courts insist that the patient be granted the right to refuse it;[50] but when he has an ineffective (non)treatment for a nondisease, he and the courts are eager to deprive the patient of his right to refuse treatment. The upshot is that psychiatrists oppose suicide that is unassisted by a physician *and* support suicide that is assisted by a physician. Physicians in general and psychiatrists in particular are ill suited, existentially as well as professionally, for the role of preventing suicide or providing assistance with it. Statistics about suicide among physicians support this view.

Preaching water but drinking wine disqualifies the speaker as a credible person and moral authority. Ophthalmologists do not go blind from untreated glaucoma more often than do lay persons. Pulmonary disease specialists do not develop emphysema more often than do lay persons. This rule holds true for all diseases except suicide. Then, physicians fail miserably: They preach suicide prevention but kill themselves more often than do lay persons: "Psychiatrists [commit] suicide, regularly, year by year, at rates about twice those expected."[51] "The suicide rate of male physicians is about three times that of the general U.S. population . . . [and] of female physi-

---

*Medical historians pare familiar with this phenomenon. The Roman medical maxim, *Primum non nocere!* (First, do no harm!) was intended as a counterweight against its enchantments.

cians at least three times that of women in the general population."[52] "Each year among the physician population, the equivalent of an average-sized medical school graduating class commits suicide."[53] Undaunted, physicians redouble their effort to hold on to the mantle of experts in suicide prevention: The House of Delegates of the American Medical Association "has voted to explore the possibility of developing a suicide-prevention program to be run by the AMA."[54]

Actions speak louder than words. The fact that physicians commit suicide more frequently than do lay persons ought to unmask their claims about suicide prevention as self-serving propaganda.

Prescribing Suicide

Death as Treatment

The only doubtful moral question on which we have to make an immediate decision in relation to involuntary euthanasia is whether we owe a moral duty to terminate the life of an insane person who is suffering from a painful and incurable disease.

—Glanville Williams (1911–1997)[1]

Incurably ill AIDS patients should be permitted to choose death as their next form of treatment.

—Canadian AIDS Society (1997)[2]

Consideration for the patient cannot be regarded as adequate ground for the necessity of destroying human life.

—Dietrich Bonhoeffer (1906–1945)[3]

Enlisting physicians in the task of killing people, whether they are patients or enemies of the State, is not a new idea. The fact that the Hippocratic Oath prohibits medical killing suggests that physicians and their superiors must have found it a temptation. The practice seems to have started in Rome under Nero: He would send "doctors to those who hesitated to execute his order to commit suicide, . . . instruct[ing] them to 'treat' (*curare*) the victims, for thus the lethal incision was called."[4] The guillotine was invented by a physician, Joseph Ignace Guillotin. The Nazi medical holocaust—the so-called euthanasia program—was planned and carried out by physicians.

The first reference in English literature to death as treatment appears in Thomas More's *Utopia* (1516). He wrote: "Should life become unbearable for these incurables, the magistrates and priests do not hesitate to prescribe euthanasia. . . . When the sick have been persuaded of this, they end their lives willingly either by starvation or drugs."[5] Not by accident, More entrusted the job of helping people to die to "magistrates and priests." In the sixteenth century, physicians lacked the prestige and social position necessary for the role. This soon changed. Francis Bacon (1561–1626) suggested that it is the physician's duty "to mitigate pain . . . not only when such mitigation may conduce to recovery, but when it may serve a fair and easy passage."[6]

In 1848, John C. Warren, the first surgeon to perform an operation using ether anesthesia, hinted that the drug might be used "in mitigating the agonies of death" and expressed the fear that it "may be employed in a criminal way, for the purpose of destroying life."[7] Ever since, many physicians and lay persons have proposed that in "cases of hopeless and painful illness, it should be the recognized duty of the medical attendant, whenever so desired by the patient, . . . [to] put the sufferer to a quick and painless death."[8]

HELPING TO DIE AS A MEDICAL MATTER

The practice of routinely referring to the ostensible beneficiary of physician-assisted suicide (PAS) as a "patient," although seemingly harmless, prejudges the act as medical and legitimizes it as beneficial ("therapeutic"). To be sure, a person dying of a terminal illness is, *ipso facto*, considered a patient. However, *dying is not a disease;* it may, *inter alia*, be a consequence of disease (or other causes, such as accident or violence). More important, *killing (oneself or someone else) is not, and by definition cannot be, a treatment.*

Language, Law, and Suicide

Advocates of PAS maintain that fatally ill patients need this service the same way that patients with acute appendicitis need an appendectomy. This is not true. A person has no *need* for another to perform a service that he could perform for himself, provided, of course, that he wants to and is allowed to perform the service for himself. If a person knows how to drive but prefers to be driven by someone else, he has no *need* for a chauffeur, he *wants* a chauffeur. Such a person is not receiving "chauffeur-assisted driving." The same is true for killing oneself. Strictly speaking, the phrase "assisted suicide" is an oxymoron.

I am not saying that medical advice and access to a lethal drug may not be helpful for committing suicide. I am saying only that autohomicide, like heterohomicide, is *not a medical matter;* it is a *legal, moral, and political matter.*[9] Neither the person who kills himself nor the physician or anyone else who gives him a lethal drug is performing a medical act. Not everything physicians do is a treatment. A physician may help another person to invest his money or improve his golf game, but that does not make these activities "treatments" (although they may figuratively be called that).

Perhaps most important, the term "physician-assisted suicide" is intrinsically mendacious: The physician is the principal, not the assistant. In the normal use of the English language, the person who assists another is the subordinate; the person whom he assists is his superior. The waiter is subordinate to the patron: he does not control what the patron orders or how much of it he eats. However, the physician engaging in PAS is superior to the patient: He determines who qualifies for the "treatment" and prescribes the drug for it.[10]

The Law is unambiguous about the issue of agency: The person in control of the operation, whether it is bank robbery or brain surgery, is the principal; his subordinate his deputy. If the act is legal, the deputy is called the "assistant"; if it is illegal, he is called the "accomplice."[11] One cannot "assist" another in murder or in any other illegal act. The person who helps another commit an illegal act is his accomplice before the fact (if he helps to plan it), during the fact (if he participates in it), or after the fact (if he tries to hide it).[12] In other words, the enterprise we call "physician-assisted suicide" is, and ought to be called, "physician-controlled suicide" or "physician-granted suicide."

We must not forget that physicians have always been partly agents of the State and are now in the process of becoming *de facto* government employees. Hence, unless a person kills himself, we cannot be certain that his death is voluntary and we ought not call the killing "suicide." Let us not forget that suicide is defined as "an act or an instance of taking one's own life voluntarily and intentionally." If a person is physically unable to kill himself and someone else kills him, then we are dealing with a clear case of heterohomicide (euthanasia or mercy killing). One of the unfortunate consequences of the controversy about physician-assisted suicide is that the false usage of the term "suicide" has become widely accepted. For example, a woman at the Memorial Sloan-Kettering Cancer Center in New York, fatally but not terminally ill, wants to die. Her friend, a veterinarian, injects a fatal dose of pentothal into her intravenous tube. The *New York Times* refers to the act as "suicide."[13] Such an act may or may not be morally wrong, juries may or may not convict the actor, but it is conceptually wrong to equate euthanasia (heterohomicide) with suicide and it is misleading to call it "suicide."

When someone else actively helps the patient, especially if he is a physician, we cannot be sure that the patient did not want to change his mind in the last moment, but could not or was not allowed to do so. We know that many persons who prepare advance directive requesting that physicians abstain from using "heroic measures" to prolong their dying change their minds when the time comes to honor their own prior requests.[14] Moreover, one of the oldest stratagems for concealing murder is making the crime scene appear as if the victim committed suicide. This possibility arises and ought to be suspected especially when a politically important person dies unexpectedly or under suspicious circumstances. Bureaucratizing PAS would make such concealment easier than it is already.

In short, conjoining the terms "assisted" and "suicide" is cognitively misleading and politically mischievous. The term "physician-assisted suicide" is a euphemism, similar to terms like "pro-choice" (for abortion) and "right to life" (for prohibiting abortion). We ought to reject PAS not only as social policy, but also as a useful term (especially so long as suicide remains, *de facto*, illegal).

Supporters and opponents of PAS alike acknowledge that *neither the Constitution nor any other American law recognizes a right to suicide*. This context frames the debate for PAS and engenders the "need" for it. If both suicide and access to drugs were *unconditionally legal*, there would be no technical need for a physician's assistance with it: People could kill themselves or could be helped to do so by family and friends. I use the phrase "unconditionally legal" to underscore that attempting suicide or being considered suicidal would not be punishable by criminal or civil (psychiatric) sanctions. I use the phrase "technical need" (the need for a surgeon's sterile gown in the operating room) to contrast it with "ceremonial need" (the need for a priest's special garb in church). Even if a person has no technical need for a physician to kill himself, he may still prefer to have such help.

However, if buying and possessing "controlled substances" without a prescription is illegal, and if only physicians have legal access to drugs, then people need to become "patients" and, as patients, need doctors to grant them access to drugs. If attempting suicide is psychiatrically illegal but becomes legal if approved by a psychiatrist, then people need to be screened by psychiatrists (for "depression") and need them as well to qualify for death by prescription. One can only marvel at the power of the cultural repression that continues to disconnect drug prohibition and CPSP from suicide. There is also a disconnect from the perceived need for legalizing physician-assisted suicide as an indirect means of letting people gain access to certain drugs (prohibited by prescription laws) and assuring them that they will not be turned into involuntary mental patients.

When (alcohol) Prohibition was the law, physicians prescribed liquor to patients who had a "medically legitimate" need for it, and people were happy to accept that evasion. Now drug prohibition is the law, physicians want to prescribe barbiturates to patients who have a "medically legitimate" need for them, and people are happy to accept that evasion. The proper remedy for Prohibition was repeal, restoring control over drinking to the citizen, not the intensified medicalization of drinking. The proper remedy for the "war on drugs" is repeal, restoring control over drug use to the citizen, not the intensified medicalization of suicide.

Finally, as long as PAS is *defined as medical treatment,* there is also a *legal need* for a physician's assistance with suicide, because a nonphysician's assistance would constitute a crime: practicing medicine without a license.

We must be careful about what we call the persons who receive and deliver suicide-assistance services. If we call the persons who receive the services "patients" and those who deliver them "physicians," then dying by means of such a service is, *ipso facto,* a "treatment," and PAS becomes an approved cause of death, like dying from a disease.* In short, the legal definition of PAS as a procedure that only a physician can perform expands the medicalization of everyday life, extends medical control over personal conduct, especially at the end of life, and diminishes patient autonomy.

Expanding the Physician's Role

In the past, physicians have helped their dying patients who are in pain by hastening their death, and people have killed themselves without the assistance of physicians. They still do. Why, then, do physicians now feel that they need laws explicitly authorizing the practice of physician-assisted suicide? Similarly, why do people now feel that they need the help of doctors to kill themselves?[15] There are at least four reasons for this: the war on drugs, fear of psychiatric punishment for failed suicide, change in the locus of death, and rejection of personal responsibility for dying voluntarily. I shall comment briefly on each, except on the fear of psychiatric punishment, which I touched on earlier.

Intensified by America's war on drugs, prescription laws effectively deprive lay persons of legally unrestricted access to most drugs, especially narcotics and sedatives, useful for relieving pain, for inducing sleep, and for committing suicide.[16] Fearing the zealous agents of the Drug Enforcement Administration (DEA), physicians are reluctant to write prescriptions for "controlled substances," especially when they suspect that the drugs may be used for suicide (or may be otherwise "abused"). These draconian prohibitions generate a demand for their medicalized evasion.

In the past, most people died at home, in a private, informal space. Now, most people die in a hospital, a public, formal space. In the home, informal rules were sufficient to regulate the dying patient's relationship with his doctor. In the hospital, the modern physician works under the glare of in-

---

*Would this make a physician's failure to kill his patient by PAS into medical negligence and a ground for a malpractice suit against him?

tense legal and professional scrutiny, requiring formal rules to regulate his relationship with patients.

Today, lay persons and physicians alike reject the proposition that the individual is personally responsible for killing himself, if that is how he wants to die, much as he is personally responsible for having children, if he wants to be a parent. Indeed, baldly stated, that proposition has become almost incomprehensible. (I discuss the reasons for this development throughout this book and especially in the last chapter.) Instead, conventional wisdom views suicide either as the tragic, preventable outcome of "untreated mental illness" or as a "right" to which dying patients are "entitled."

In short, we systematically criminalize, medicalize, and politicize both drugs and suicide and generate ever-increasing dependence on the medical profession to prescribe drugs for all manner of human problems unrelated to diseases. This, in turn, leads to defining ever more nondiseases as diseases, ever more ordinary human acts as treatments, and to ever more measures as "protections" of people from "abuses."

The federal Controlled Substances Act specifies that, to be lawful, a prescription for a controlled substance "must be issued for a *legitimate medical purpose* by an individual practitioner acting *in the usual course of his professional practice.* . . . An order purporting to be a prescription issued *not in the usual course of professional treatment* . . . is *not a prescription* within the meaning and intent of section 309 of the Act."[17] It follows that, to bring PAS into conformity with the requirements of this act, *writing a prescription for a lethal drug as a medical treatment must be defined as a treatment.*

The motivations for demanding physician-assisted suicide are symmetrical: Physicians are rightly afraid of the Drug Enforcement Administration (that is, being punished for prescribing "controlled substances" in violation of explicit DEA policy) and want to be reassured that they will not be so punished in cases of PAS. Patients are rightly afraid of psychiatry (that is, becoming the victims of coercive psychiatry) and want to be reassured that they will be spared this fate if they try to kill themselves and fail. Also, patients fear what I call "the fatal temptation," that is, yielding to the lure of easy suicide with drugs, and thus conspire in their own loss of liberty.[18] Finally, the physicians' and patients' needs and demands for PAS mesh with the interest of the State to bring ever more aspects of personal conduct under medical control and threaten to further strengthen the Therapeutic State.

COMPASSION IN DYING V. STATE OF WASHINGTON

McNaghten[19] is a landmark case in the legal history of the insanity defense. *Roe v. Wade*[20] is a landmark case in the legal history of abortion. *Compassion in Dying v. State of Washington* (CDW)[21] is likely to become a landmark case in the legal history of PAS. A brief review of this case is necessary for an understanding of the legal realities concerning PAS.*

Compassion in Dying, the principal plaintiff in the case, is a private, nonprofit organization established in 1993, ostensibly to defend the cause of "dying patients" from needless suffering by offering them the option of physician-assisted suicide.[22]† Joined by four physicians, Compassion in Dying brought suit against the State of Washington, seeking a declaration by the court that the statutes that prohibit "causing or aiding another person to commit suicide violate the Federal Constitution." The plaintiffs claimed that: (1) Physicians have a constitutionally protected right to assist terminally ill suicidal patients by giving them a prescription for a lethal drug. (2) Terminally ill patients have a constitutionally protected right to receive PAS. (3) PAS is a *bona fide* medical treatment.

The claim that PAS is a "treatment" was also advanced in the closely related case of *Quill v. Vacco*, where plaintiffs declared: "[Writing] a prescription [for a lethal drug], which only a licensed medical doctor can provide . . . is a complex medical task."[23] Under the guise of increasing patient autonomy, physicians, allied with the State, are once again trying to increase their power over the laity. The strategy of medicalizing laws governing suicide closely parallels the strategies of medicalizing the laws governing drug use.

The U.S. District Court for the Western District of Washington granted summary judgment for the plaintiffs. The State appealed. On March 6, 1996, the U. S. Court of Appeals for the Ninth Circuit held "that provision of the statute that prohibited aiding another person to commit suicide violated due process clause as applied to *terminally ill patients* who wished to hasten their own deaths *with medication prescribed by their physician.*"[24] The majority opinion, written by Circuit Judge Stephen Reinhardt, began with a passionate restatement of a "woman's right to an abortion"; continued with vignettes of the plaintiff-patients—each of whom was said to have wished "to commit suicide by taking physician-prescribed drugs"—(who had died by the time the ruling was handed down); and concluded with the declaration: "In deciding right-to-die cases, we are guided by the [Supreme] Court's approach to the abortion cases. . . . [In *Roe v. Wade*] the Court

---

*The complete text runs to 69 pages and contains 161 footnotes. The majority opinion contains many observations and comments about abortion, terminating lifesupport, and suicide. Its length and breadth make the judges' silence on the role of drug laws in suicide all the more deafening.

†Limiting PAS to terminally ill patients was only a part of the organization's foot-in-the-door tactic. In December 1997, a fund-raising letter declared: "We have expanded our mission to include not only terminally ill individuals, but also persons with incurable illnesses which will *eventually* lead to a terminal diagnosis."

determined that women had a liberty interest in securing abortions."[25] *Ergo*, terminally ill patients have a liberty interest in securing PAS.

Not so. Formerly, the desire to end the life of a healthy fetus was defined as a disease that affected the pregnant woman, and therapeutic abortion on psychiatric grounds was defined as a treatment for that disease. Now, the desire to end one's own life is defined as a disease and, depending on the circumstances, coercive psychiatric suicide *and* physician-assisted suicide are defined as treatments for them. I maintain that incarcerating a depressed person to prevent him from killing himself, writing a prescription for a terminally ill patient, and aborting the healthy fetus of a healthy woman are procedures we accept as legally permissible *medical interventions, but they are not medical treatments*, because the conditions they "treat" are not diseases. Each is an instance of self-deception and social deception in the interest of evading personal responsibility and/or legal prohibition.

The analogy between abortion and suicide is misleading. Abortion is heterohomicide, whereas suicide is autohomicide. Physicians successfully treat the diseases of four-month-old fetuses in utero.[26] Pregnant women who smoke crack have been successfully prosecuted for endangering the welfare of their children and for involuntary manslaughter.[27] I cite these facts not as arguments against abortion (which is another subject), but to underscore that abortion belongs to an altogether different moral category than does suicide. Also, abortion typically requires the *technical* assistance of a physician, but suicide does not.

After reviewing past and present social attitudes toward suicide, the judges emphasized that granting terminally ill patients a "right to die" does not imply granting people a right to suicide. On the contrary, they re-emphasized that it is the duty of the State to prevent suicide:

The fact that neither Washington nor any other state currently bans suicide, or attempted suicide, does not mean that the state does not have a valid and important interest in preventing or discouraging the act. . . . *The state has a clear interest in preventing anyone, no matter what age, from taking his own life in a fit of desperation, depression, or loneliness or as a result of any other problem, physical or psychological, which can be significantly ameliorated.* Studies show that many suicides are committed by people who are suffering from *treatable mental disorders*. Most if not all states provide for the involuntary commitment of such persons if they are likely to physically harm themselves.[28]

Note, however, that the right to SP and the right to PAS are mutually contradictory. Everyone classified as "terminally ill" *ipso facto* has a physical problem that can be "significantly ameliorated," and anyone who contemplates suicide is considered "likely to physically harm himself."

The method judges use to distinguish persons "likely to physically harm themselves" from those not likely to do so is also troublesome: They do so by listening to doctors. Different physicians may tell different things to different judges. What physicians tell judges may or may not be true. Even if what they tell judges is true, the judges' ignorance of medicine may render them unable to understand it. This possibility is starkly illustrated by the judges' blunder in CDW. Observing that individuals intent on killing themselves but "deprived of physician assistance" may resort to desperate methods, the judges cite the case of "a terminally ill patient [who] took his own life by withholding his insulin and letting himself die of insulin shock [sic]."[29] The judges' unfamiliarity with the elementary difference between diabetic coma and insulin shock does not bode well for their monitoring PAS.

Similarly, Oregon's Death with Dignity Act (DWDA) "relies on the physician's clinical judgment" to assess the patient's eligibility to receive a lethal prescription and specifies that *"No judicial hearing is required."*[30] The absence of judicial hearing as a condition for PAS hardly comports with the requirements of the Rule of Law.

Moreover, the physician who performs physician-assisted suicide does not merely render a clinical judgment and perform a medical intervention; he also renders a moral judgment and performs a social ritual. He legitimizes PAS as *not irrational* and therefore not wrong, exactly as he illegitimizes physician-unassisted suicide as *irrational* and therefore wrong; and he *defines* prescribing a lethal drug as a *therapeutic response to a medical crisis* rather than as a *pseudomedical evasion of drug prohibition*, exactly as he *defines* involuntary mental hospitalization as a *therapeutic response to dangerousness due to mental disease* rather than as a *pseudomedical deprivation of liberty*.

In June 1997, the U.S. Supreme Court, by a vote of 9 to 0, upheld State laws prohibiting assisted suicide.[31] "Our decision," wrote Chief Justice William H. Rehnquist, "leads us to conclude that the asserted 'right' to assistance in committing suicide is not a fundamental liberty interest protected by the due-process clause."[32]

PAS, Drugs, and the Principle of Double Effect

Western Law and Medicine have long approved of physicians giving terminally ill patients drugs whose effect is to hasten the patient's death, a practice justified by the principle of "double effect."[33] Advocates of PAS try to justify that practice by appealing to this familiar principle. However, the essential act in PAS differs radically from the essential act in traditional physician-aided death.

When we speak of the double effect of a drug that the physician gives to terminally ill patients, we refer typically to morphine (an analgesic) being *administered* by a doctor to a *helpless patient for the relief of suffering.* However, when we speak of the double effect of a drug used for physician-assisted suicide, we refer typically to a barbiturate (a soporific) which the doctor *prescribes for a patient who is not helpless and which he "ingests on his own" to kill himself.*[34] Barbiturates are not pain killers, and the only reason the doctor prescribes a lethal dose of the drug is to enable the patient to kill himself with it. Ignoring these differences, the majority opinion in CDW states: "[W]e see little, if any, difference for constitutional or ethical purposes between providing medication with a double effect and providing medication with a single effect, as long as one of the known effects in each case is to hasten the end of the patient's life."[35] We may deem such medical behavior morally praiseworthy or blameworthy, but we cannot maintain that the principle of double effect applies, "for constitutional purposes," to the action of a drug ingested for the express purpose of killing oneself.

The judges further assert that they see "no ethically or constitutionally cognizable difference between a doctor's pulling the plug on a respirator and his prescribing drugs which will permit a terminally ill patient to end his own life. . . . To the extent that a difference exists, we conclude that it is one of degree and not of kind."[36] This, too, is erroneous. A respirator enables a patient to breathe when he cannot breathe on his own. Disconnecting the respirator lets the patient *die of the disease.* Prescribing a lethal drug for a patient who wants to kill himself lets the patient *die of self-killing.* Not prescribing a lethal drug results in the patient not dying when he wants to die (which is why he wants the prescription). The moral and legal difference between *assisting* a person to kill himself and *desisting* from keeping him alive against his will is quintessentially a difference of kind, not of degree.

Holding that suicide is wrongful, the advocates of PAS feel compelled to redefine the meaning of the word "suicide." Circuit Judge Stephen Reinhardt and his colleagues write: "We are doubtful that deaths resulting from terminally ill patients taking *medication prescribed by their doctors* should be classified as 'suicide'."[37] Oregon's DWDA advances the same claim: "Actions taken in accordance with this Act shall not, for any purpose, constitute suicide, assisted suicide, mercy killing, or homicide."[38] How can physician-assisted suicide not be suicide or assisted suicide when those terms form a part of the phrase by which everyone calls the act?

Classifying PAS as not suicide transforms the act into an abstraction, the impersonal consequence of the double effect, originally a theological dodge, now a bioethical evasion. Physician-assisted suicide thus becomes an event for which nothing and no one is responsible. That is one of the things that makes it so appealing to people fleeing responsibility in general and responsibility for suicide in particular.

PAS, Abortion, and Mental Illness

As we have seen, one of the justifications advanced for a right to PAS is the alleged analogy between it and a right to abortion. This is misleading, partly for reasons noted above and partly for other reasons, discussed below. Advocates for PAS insist that candidates for the procedure be screened by psychiatrists for mental illness, especially depression (against the patient's will if necessary). Columbia University psychiatrist Philip R. Muskin writes: "[Legislation] should *require* that doctors explore why their patients have requested to die. In cases where it is appropriate, the law should *require* that doctors consult with a psychiatrist to evaluate the patient's request."[39]

Thirty years ago, when abortion was illegal, advocates of physician-assisted abortion claimed that the most common indication for a therapeutic abortion (TA) was depression and the risk of suicide. To secure a TA, the pregnant woman had only to claim that she was depressed, would rather kill herself than have the baby, and would pay for the service.[40*] Unless she made such a threat, she was deemed ineligible for a TA on psychiatric grounds. Women who requested a TA and made such threats were, of course, not subjected to psychiatric screening or involuntary psychiatric treatment, nor were they forced to endure the biological consequences of their condition (pregnancy). Yet, the advocates for PAS propose imposing precisely these requirements and consequences on dying patients: They repeat *ad nauseam* that the procedure ought to be limited to nondepressed patients and that depressed dying patients be subjected to involuntary psychiatric treatment and compelled to endure the biological consequences of their condition (dying from their illness).

Why did advocates for psychiatric-therapeutic abortion not try to restrict the procedure to nondepressed women? Because they considered being depressed an appropriate reaction for a pregnant woman who does not want to have a baby and must beg for an abortion, and they believed that it would have been an insult to expect that such a woman not be depressed. Similar considerations apply to dying patients who request PAS. It is an insult to expect that such a person not be depressed. Pieter V. Admiraal, a prominent figure in the Dutch euthanasia movement, agrees: "To send a terminally ill patient to a psychiatrist is an insult." Admiraal dismisses, as self-serving, the doctors who "say that . . . requesting euthanasia must be the result of depression and will prescribe antidepressant drugs."[41]

It seems improbable that the court in *Roe v. Wade* simply forgot to limit the right to abortion to nondepressed women. More likely, the judges ac-

---

*Because patients had to pay for therapeutic abortions, this option was generally foreclosed to poor women.

cepted depression as an appropriate mental state for a pregnant woman who wants an abortion but who must convince a physician to perform the procedure. Similarly, judges who analogize PAS to TA ought to accept depression as an appropriate mental state for a dying patient who wants to kill himself with a drug but must convince a physician to prescribe it for him. This statement is not intended as an endorsement of the practice. I do not believe in a "right" to physician-assisted suicide, partly because I believe that if people could access drugs without obstruction by physicians and the law, PAS would be a nonissue, and partly because the concept of right implies reciprocal obligations.[42]

In short, the appeal to this false analogy between physician-assisted suicide and therapeutic abortion is deeply disturbing. Although in each case the diagnosis of depression functions as a medico-legal tactic, in the case of TA, depression justifies *providing* the intervention requested by the patient, whereas in the case of PAS, it justifies *withholding* it. Moreover, legalizing abortion eliminated the need for women to "beg" for the procedure and for physicians to pretend that it is medically necessary; whereas legalizing PAS would not eliminate the need for dying patients to beg for lethal drugs nor for physicians to pretend that it is medically necessary. On the contrary, legalizing PAS would intensify these needs by further authenticating the wisdom of drug prohibition and the illusion that when doctors bootleg lethal drugs they are treating patients.

MEDICAL KILLING IS NOT MERCY KILLING*

The term "mercy killing" conjures up the image of a veterinarian putting an old dog "to sleep" or a John Wayne—six-shooter in hand, sun blazing in the desert sky, vultures circling overhead—administering the *coup de grace* to his faithful horse with a broken leg. Professing compassion for suffering patients, advocates of PAS exclaim: "You wouldn't let an animal die like this." This is propaganda for medical killing. It tells us nothing about suicide. The analogy between physician-assisted suicide and the mercy killing of a moribund pet is deceptive. Animals cannot commit suicide. Medical execution, however merciful, is not suicide.

Mercy Killing Must Be Personal, Not Bureaucratic

On the face of it, there seems to be nothing morally objectionable about helping a beloved relative or friend kill himself if he asks for such help and if we consider his decision to be sound. However, approving of such an act

---

*The English word "mercy" comes from, and is the same as, the French "*merci*." Today, *merci* means "thanks," but originally it meant forberarance to someone in one's power.

does not support the case for legalizing PAS. As a private, personal act, helping a relative or friend kill himself may be laudable. It does not follow that it is therefore also laudable to bureaucratize suicide assistance and define it as a treatment, to restrict its practice to physicians, and to authorize doctors to restrict the treatment to persons formally diagnosed as terminally ill and free of mental illness.

My colleague Robert Daly offered the following example to illustrate the fundamental differences between personal and professional assistance with suicide. Jack, a soldier retreating from the front, finds his buddy, Jim, mortally wounded. In great pain but lucid, Jim asks Jack for the *coup de grace*. Jack complies. Daly concludes: "It is difficult for me to declare this request and compliance with it 'immoral.' It is difficult to discern the goods that are secured and the evils avoided by requiring in the name of morality that the mortally wounded soldier be required to cling to his life, especially when he is legally required to sacrifice that life for the good of our country."[43]

Daly's point is that we do not regard Jack's killing Jim as part of his role as a soldier. If Jack complies with Jim's request, he is helping Jim as buddy, not as soldier. Daly concludes: "Even if there are acceptable reasons for not finding all suicides morally wrong, or assistance by others in these acts permissible, a physician, simply because she is a physician, assisting in ending life [especially that of the physician's patient] is simply and always socially imprudent if not morally evil."[44]

Relatives, friends, and physicians have always helped, and still help, aged and sick persons to die. They did it, and do it, quietly and in private. How often they did it or do it now no one knows. The point is that as long as such aid-in-dying entails neither force nor fraud and does not visibly violate mores and laws, it remains a private affair, willingly overlooked by the authorities. However, when killing is defined as a type of healing, as a specialized professional role, then the legal apparatus of the State takes a keen interest in it, as well it should. Policemen, executioners, and soldiers are authorized by the State to kill certain domestic and foreign enemies, under certain circumstances. Physicians are authorized by the State to practice medicine. Medical licensure entails, among other things, granting doctors special powers, for example, to prevent suicide:

- The State authorizes physicians to make an exception to the rule that innocent persons have a constitutional right to liberty: Psychiatrists *select* certain individuals as qualifying for involuntary mental hospitalization *in their own best medical interest.*

Advocates for a right to PAS want to extend these privileges. They believe that:

- The State ought to authorize physicians to make exceptions to the rule that prohibits them from prescribing drugs except for the treatment or alleviation of disease: They ought to be able to *select* certain individuals as qualifying to receive a
  prescription for a lethal drug, *in their own best medical interest.*

One must be blind not to see that such a policy defines the physician as a superior and the patient as a subordinate and that it must inexorably result in
further diminishing personal autonomy, liberty, and responsibility.

Because American proposals for PAS restrict the procedure to persons
able to self-administer the prescribed drug, patients too disabled to do so
would be excluded from its benefits. Advocates for PAS argue that this is
unfair. Perhaps it is. However, if the patient does not self-administer the
drug, then the intervention ought to be called "medical killing" or "mercy
killing," not suicide. After that threshold is crossed, another thorny problem is sure to arise; namely, how to distinguish persons who cannot kill
themselves because they are in fact unable to do so from persons who could
kill themselves and only pretend to be unable to do so to qualify for PAS.

This is an important distinction. If a person can kill himself but chooses
not to do so and, instead, asks a physician to kill him, then the help he receives is like that of a child who can tie his shoelaces but asks his parent to
tie them for him. Impatient, the parent may comply. We do not call that
compassion; we call it convenience. The same thing is likely to happen in
the case of PAS. For obvious reasons, patients and physicians alike may prefer PAS to PUS (physician-unassisted suicide). This is a cause for concern
for many reasons, not least because these are situations unregulated by the
constraints intrinsic to market relations: Prominent advocates for PAS are
in alarming agreement about rejecting selling the service for money. This
may make the merchants of death seem like disinterested philanthropists,
but it leaves unanswered the question of why would any *physician qua physician* want to engage in the practice. Physicians receive payment for the
services they render, if not from the patient directly then from someone else
or the State. And patients ought to know that, as Shakespeare put it, "You
pay a great deal too dear for what's given freely."[45]

The benefit the parent who ties his child's shoelaces receives is saving
time and avoiding unpleasantness. What benefit does the physician who
provides "suicide assistance" expect to receive in exchange for his services?
As a rule, the enthusiast eager to help the Other not for money but for a
cause is driven by a desire for the rewards of "existential cannibalism," that
is, sucking meaning (admiration, excitement, fame) out of the misery of his
beneficiaries.[46] All history teaches us that, especially in relations between
competent adults unrelated by strong bonds of family or friendship, if the
recipient does not pay for the service he receives, it is likely that the service
he gets is *not* the service he wants. Examining the words and deeds of the

two most prominent American doctors of death, Jack Kevorkian and Timothy E. Quill, provides more specific information about why they advocate death as a treatment.

DR. JACK KEVORKIAN: OBITIATRIST

Jack Kevorkian, a former pathologist, has become famous for helping scores of persons commit "suicide." Although he flaunts his contempt for PAS as unworthy of the physician's concerns, the media have so misrepresented his views that, in the popular mind, he has become one of the leading advocates for PAS.[47]

Medicide and Obitiatry

In *Prescription: Medicide,* Kevorkian emphasizes that his "ultimate aim [is] not simply to help suffering or doomed persons to kill themselves—that is merely the first step, an early distasteful professional obligation (now called medicide) that nobody in his or her right mind could savor. . . . [W]hat I find most satisfying is the prospect of making possible the performance of invaluable experiments or other beneficial acts . . . in a word, obitiatry."[48] The term "medicide" is typical of Kevorkian's inept neologisms. As germicide means killing germs, so medicide means, or ought to mean, killing medicine or killing doctors.

Obitiatry, Kevorkian further explains, "is the name of the medical specialty concerned with the treatment or doctoring of death to achieve some sort of beneficial result, in the same way that psychiatry is the name of the medical specialty concerned with the treatment or doctoring of the psyche for the beneficial result of mental health."[49] According to Kevorkian, death is "doctored," not patients; the doctoring is done by obitiatry, not by doctors; and the subject's death is caused by a machine (the "Mercitron"), not a person:

[N]o longer is there a need—or even an excuse—for anyone to be the direct mediator of the death of another who is alert, rational, and who for some compelling reason chooses to, or must, die. Performance of that repulsive task should now be relegated exclusively to a device like the Mercitron, which the doomed subject must activate. . . . [M]*edicide has now been eliminated as an ethical problem for the medical profession*. . . . The device's impact on morality extends to execution chambers as well. . . . Only by using the Mercitron . . . [can] the execution be made even more humane. . . . The Mercitron can diffuse it [moral guilt] even more by *eliminating entirely the need for anyone to inject anything*.[50]

By attributing self-killing to mental illness, the psychiatrist eliminates the mental patient as a moral agent responsible for his act . Similarly, by at-

tributing killing the "doomed person" to the Mercitron, Kevorkian eliminates both the physician and the subject as moral agents responsible for
their actions. Obitiatrists and psychiatrists both oppose "irrational" suicide: "For the first time in history, medicide would offer the objective means
of *distinguishing rational from irrational suicide*. After all, with that option at
hand, would anyone in his or her right mind 'choose' (that is, driven by
panic) instead to commit suicide by other ordinary, messy, and usually violent means?"[51]

Kevorkian identifies himself with his Armenian forebears murdered in
the Turkish holocaust, yet glamorizes physician-participation in State-
sponsored killing, crediting the practice to medieval Armenian scientists:
"Criminals condemned to death in medieval Armenia were vivisected for
the purpose of not only studying the complexity of human anatomy, but
also searching for better ways of treating and preventing disease."[52]
Kevorkian concludes: "The time is not far off when the culling of medical
benefit [sic], too, from rationally planned death will denote the highest degree of morality applied to the legal and purposeful termination of individual human lives. . . . In short, *medical experimentation on consenting humans
was, is, and most likely always will be a laudable and correct thing to do.*"[53]

Kevorkian on Suicide

We use the word "suicide" to refer to voluntary (noncoerced) self-
killing. Kevorkian uses it to denote the following types of killings:

Obligatory Assisted Suicide. This includes everyone who must, without exception or
recourse, be put to death by a person or agency having sole jurisdiction over killing.
. . . [T]he executioners may or may not be legitimately empowered. . . . *Optional Assisted Suicide*. This is for those individuals . . . who choose to be killed by another as
the preferable of only two almost equally unpleasant alternatives. . . . [Such as] the
forebears of Christianity in ancient Rome. . . . *Obligatory Suicide*. . . . The ritual suicide
of *suttee* in India . . . fits this category. . . . *Optional Suicide*. For persons who are in no
way afflicted by illness but have arbitrarily and irrevocably decided that they must
die. . . . *Suicide by Proxy*. This category encompasses the killing, by the decision and
action of another, of fetuses, infants, minor children, and every human being incapable of giving direct informed consent.[54]

Abortion, infanticide, judicially authorized execution, and gangland
killing are all instances of "suicide." Satisfied with that classification,
Kevorkian states: "The above list of categories encompasses all potential
candidates for the *humane killing known as euthanasia, by others or the self.*"[55]
Despite his clearly expressed opposition to suicide and support for involuntary medical killing, many people think that Kevorkian defends the indi-

vidual's right to suicide. A psychologist even identifies him as an "exponent of Hume's position."[56]

To the press and the public, Kevorkian represents his activities as a medical obligation. He tells a reporter for the *Detroit News*: "There was a patient suffering. . . . I'm a physician. . . . My duty is to this patient."[57] However, Kevorkian is not, and never was, a *practicing physician*. He was a pathologist. His "subjects" were cadavers. By the time he began to practice obitiatry, he was a *retired* pathologist. Kevorkian maintains that because he has a medical degree, he has a right to help suffering patients commit suicide; that suffering patients have a right to suicide with his assistance; and that he does not help anyone to commit suicide. In one of his court appearances, his lawyer, Geoffrey Fieger, asked him: " 'Have you ever wanted a patient to die?' 'Never,' Kevorkian said."[58] In another court appearance, Kevorkian "branded his accuser, the Oakland County prosecutor Richard Thompson, 'a lying psychotic' . . . [and] denied 'he has ever assisted in a suicide.' " Fieger, too, maintains that "all Kevorkian does is 'engage in the relief of human suffering.' . . . 'I am not aware that he [Kevorkian] has ever been present at any suicide. He has sometimes been present when people have ended their horrific suffering.' "[59]

As the number of suicides acknowledged to have occurred in Kevorkian's "presence" increased, the press lost interest in him. In June 1998, in an evident bid for fresh publicity, Kevorkian enacted the dream he had announced in *Medicide*, "the culling of medical benefit . . . from rationally planned death."[60] After helping a 45-year-old quadriplegic man to die, unnamed person or persons removed the man's kidneys, and Kevorkian offered them to any transplantation team that wanted them.[61] None did.

DR. TIMOTHY E. QUILL: THE DOCTOR WITH THE "SILKY MANNERS"

Timothy E. Quill is professor of medicine *and* psychiatry at the University of Rochester. Long before Quill appeared on the scene, C. S. Lewis warned about the coming of the type of medical persona to which Quill aspires. "The new Nero," wrote Lewis, "will approach us with the silky manners of a doctor, and though all will in fact be compulsory . . . all will go on within the unemotional therapeutic sphere where words like 'right' and 'wrong' or 'freedom' and 'slavery' are never heard."[62]

Reluctant Zealot: Death as "Self-Preservation"

In a legal case that bears his name, *Quill v. Vacco*, Quill sued the State of New York, ostensibly on behalf of patients, asking that it formally authorize physicians to help certain patients commit suicide: "Terminally ill persons who seek to hasten death by consuming drugs need medical counseling . . . as well as a prescription, which only a licensed medical doctor can provide. . . . [Performing this service] is a complex medical task."[63]

Like Kevorkian, Quill disdains PAS. He tells a reporter: "I am not really an advocate of assisted suicide. I am an advocate of not abandoning people."[64] The district attorney for Monroe County (in Rochester, New York) loves this pretense which saves him from having to prosecute Quill and praises him for "not embarking on a crusade . . . or to get publicity for himself." This is far from true. A reporter correctly observes that Quill "did launch something of a crusade. . . . [He] challenged the New York law that bans assisted suicide. . . . The case neatly summarizes Quill's belief that writing a lethal prescription is morally and ethically equivalent to unplugging a respirator."[65]

Quill is careful to distance himself from the image of the doctor as killer. In his book, *A Midwife Through the Dying Process*, he calls himself a midwife to the dying patient and writes: "The best way to get beneath the surface of the personal and ethical challenges of dying is through real-life patient narratives." However, Quill's stories are *not* "patient narratives." They are "physician narratives," the narrator being Quill himself. The stories are simply *his version* of nine "cases." Although Quill asserts his devotion to patients, he violates the most elementary requirements of a decent doctor-patient relationship: He is intrusive, patronizing, and confuses controlling the patient with caring for him: "The wish to die demands exploration," Quill's euphemism for psychiatric meddling defined as "care."[66] The wish not to die, albeit mortally ill, evidently does not demand "exploration."

Quill maintains that his relationship to his patients is a "partnership": "Partnership and nonabandonment are the core obligations of humane medical care for the dying."[67] Quill's idea of partnership is elastic: It allows him to turn the patient's misery into a "case history" without the patient's permission. He acknowledges that in some of the cases, "permission was granted by families, *who believed their loved ones would want their story to be told*."[68] That is an unpersuasive excuse. Calling the patients' deaths "good" and "life affirming" is not a substitute for their informed consent.[69] Quill's patients did not die suddenly. He had time enough to obtain permission from them. He did not.

Quill is an enthusiast for the psychiatric assessment and reassessment of dying patients, even when such meddling is clearly inimical to the patient's self-declared wishes. One of his patients wanted his defibrillator deactivated. According to Quill, he was "not clinically depressed" and had "an accurate grasp of his medical condition and prognosis."[70] Nevertheless, the patient was evaluated by psychiatrists, as if they could have distinguished between his being "clinically depressed" and being just plain depressed because of his medical condition. "There are," Quill adds in a rare moment of candor, "no fully agreed upon standards of rationality and competence for making these types of medical decisions."[71] Instead of rejecting psychiatric meddling in the lives of dying persons, Quill advocates *more* such meddling, not because it helps the patients, but because "Unraveling the potential contribution of depression [to wanting to die] can be challenging."[72]

At the core of Quill's words and deeds lies the patently false, self-serving premise that dying is a "medical emergency." He writes: "[When] dying becomes dominated by disintegration, it is nothing short of a medical emergency."[73] Dying *is* disintegration. But dying *slowly* is not an emergency, although Quill insists that it may be: "These few bad deaths [of patients who supposedly cannot be made comfortable] must be considered a *medical emergency*. People sometimes end up in very bad situations at the end of life, and you have to be creative, bold, in the way you help them. . . . [Y]ou solve what has to be solved."[74] To a reporter for *Newsweek*, he explains: "I don't see this [PAS] as suicide. These people feel their self is being destroyed by their illness. They view death as a form of self-preservation."[75] Fittingly, the caption under Quill's picture reads: "Death as self-preservation: Dr. Timothy Quill."

Dying may be many things, but it cannot be a "medical emergency," a term that refers to a patient who would die without prompt and appropriate medical intervention, but who would probably live if given such "life-saving" help. Thus, the situation of a patient who, regardless of medical intervention, is certain to die and will probably die soon cannot, by definition, constitute a medical emergency.

Historically, the term "emergency" has been indispensable in the lexicon of the tyrant masquerading as therapist. Madison warned: "Crisis is the rallying cry of the tyrant."[76] The politician who wants to suspend the constraints of the rule of law cries "national emergency." Dutch doctors, as we shall see, justify both voluntary euthanasia (VE) *and* involuntary euthanasia by postulating a "concept of the state of emergency within which the physician acts."[77] Physicians anxious to reject the constraints of cooperation and contract with the patient, exemplified by Quill and psychiatrists in general, cry "medical emergency."

Although Quill presents himself as an ordinary doctor, a modern version of the family physician, he is also a psychiatrist. Taking for granted that suicide is a medical problem, he writes: "Whenever a severely ill person begins to talk about wanting to die . . . the question of clinical depression appropriately arises. This can be a complex and delicate determination because most patients who are near death with unrelenting suffering are very sad, if not clinically depressed."[78] The only reason such a hypothetical patient would be in a state of "unrelenting suffering" is because of prevailing drug policies, endorsed by psychiatrists like Quill, eager to increase the physician's prescription-writing privileges and powers. Avoiding reference to coercive suicide prevention, Quill cautions: "Sometimes the wish for death is a cry for help.... At other times it is indicative of clinical depression darkly distorting one's perceptions, perhaps amenable to psychotherapy or antidepressant medication."[79]

The Mask of Responsibility

The most important justification for making suicide assistance a *medical* intervention, according to Quill, is "the loneliness and abandonment of the patient at death. This is perhaps the most serious flaw in the current system. . . . [O]ur laws say that . . . if you die by suicide you have to be alone. To me that is unacceptable."[80]

That is an argument for involving family and friends in voluntary death, not for giving more power to physicians. Socrates did not die alone. He was assisted by his friends and pupils, not by physicians. Quill ignores all nonmedical options of suicide assistance and proposes, instead, that the physician be Lady Bountiful, keeping the dying patient "therapeutic company." However, as long as the suicide-assisting physician possesses power not only to facilitate the subject's voluntary death, but also to foil it by incarcerating him in a mental hospital, this is an abhorrent proposal.

We should beware of Quill's cant about "assuming responsibility" for his patients, a phrase superiors typically use to conceal their desire to control their subordinates. Masters were responsible for their slaves. Parents are responsible for their minor children. Accused of authorizing the circumcision of his daughter, a Somali father in Houston, Texas, explained: "It's my responsibility. If I don't do it, I will have failed my children."[81]

Quill's "silky manners" appeal to many people, especially liberals who see domineering doctors as benevolent healers. Arguing the case for PAS before the Supreme Court, Harvard Law Professor Laurence Tribe characterized Quill as "a good representative of what ought to happen."[82] Quill's critics, of which there are many, see him as exhibiting, in Daniel Callahan's words, "lethal sentimentality."[83] Richard Doerflinger, associate director for policy at the Secretariat for Pro-Life Activities of the National Conference of Catholic Bishops, states: "In some ways, Dr. Quill is even more extreme than Dr. Kevorkian: he defends direct lethal injections by physicians and has praised a ruling by the Ninth Circuit Court of Appeals that authorizes 'surrogates' to order lethal drugs for incompetent patients who never asked for death."[84] Michael McQuillen, professor of neurology at Quill's medical school, observes: "They [Kevorkian and Quill] both are accomplishing the same end, the one with a hacksaw, and the other with a fine surgeon's knife."[85]

THE DEBATE ABOUT PAS AND VE

Instead of confronting the moral and legal dilemmas posed by our policies regulating drug use and suicide, the press, professionals, and the public take sides for or against PAS. As a result, much of the current commentary about physician-assisted suicide and voluntary euthanasia is a distraction; it diverts attention from the problems posed by two sets of interlocking ideas and practices: "dangerous drugs" and drug laws, on the one hand, "dangerousness to self and others" and mental health laws, on the other hand. Critical debate is inhibited by what is, in effect, a social taboo—a conspiracy of silence—regarding drug policy and suicide policy as *moral and legal issues* in their own right and as policies *logically anterior to policies about PAS and VE as medical procedures.* Being accepted as a respected contributor to the debate about PAS requires respecting the taboo against linking it with the war on drugs and CPSP. An editorial in the *New York Times*, published two days before the Supreme Court's scheduled hearing on PAS, is illustrative:

This page has argued that terminally ill, mentally competent adults nearing death should have the option of dying with dignity, in full control of their bodies and final moments. With others who share that view, we hope the Court will see clearly the profoundly important issue of personal liberty that lies at the controversy's core. A wise decision would recognize both the rights of suffering terminally ill patients and the duty of states to craft safeguards to prevent abuse.[86]

PAS and VE: Professionals, the Press, and the Public

Supporters of PAS and VE base their case largely on the analogy between refusing treatment and prescribing a lethal drug, and on the contention that giving physicians more "therapeutic" discretion and power increases the autonomy and dignity of patients. The following statement is typical: "[T]here is essentially no difference between the permissible withdrawal of essential nutrition, hydration, respiration, kidney dialysis or other treatment that is artificially prolonging life and the prescribing of drugs that would allow a dying patient who is suffering intolerably a humane death within his or her own control. . . . The Court has an obligation to cut through the contrived reasoning behind laws and practices that deny dignity and personal autonomy at the end of life."[87]

The writer's selective indignation is a poor substitute for reasoning. He considers denying drugs to dying patients who want to kill themselves as a violation of their personal autonomy, but he evidently does not consider denying drugs to responsible, hard-working citizens a violation of their personal autonomy. He considers killing oneself under conditions approved by physicians and with their assistance a constitutional right, but he evidently considers killing oneself when one wants to without physician assistance a mental illness and violation of the mental health laws. This mantra has replaced meaningful dialogue.

In 1996, when the Supreme Court was considering the case of *Compassion in Dying v. State of Washington*, the Newark (NJ) diocese of the Episcopal Church filed an *amicus curiae* brief supporting the right to PAS.[88] David Bird, rector of Grace Church in Georgetown in Washington, DC, and vice chair of the Medical Ethics Committee of the Episcopal Diocese of Washington, declared: "There is no divine imperative upon us to prolong dying . . . I believe, therefore, that in appropriate circumstances God would rather endorse our Christian moral courage in actively participating in assisting the suicide of certain terminally ill patients."[89] He also lamented that "We are apparently maintaining biological existence to no *human purpose*. . . . More than 10,000 American adults remain in nursing homes and hospitals in vegetative comas with no hope of recovery, at the public cost of $350,000,000 each year."[90]

Richard Westley, professor of philosophy at Chicago's Loyola University (a Catholic institution), sees divine warrant for VE: "It is my basic assumption," he writes, "that there is a divine revelation about death that is not being heeded. . . . The question of who should perform the act of euthanasia is ultimately the most difficult and agonizing question we have to face. . . . The decision should be made by a consensus of the patient, health care personnel, family, friends, and the patient's religious shepherd."[91] For Westley, the moral problem is not whether euthanasia is licit or not, but who decides who should perform it.

Derek Humphry, the founder of the Hemlock Society, is widely regarded as an advocate of the right to suicide. He is not. His organization, revealingly called Euthanasia Research & Guidance Organization (ERGO), is dedicated to the proposition that there are two radically different kinds of suicide. Humphry explains: "One is 'emotional suicide,' or irrational self-murder. . . . ERGO's view of this tragic form of self-destruction is the same as that of the *suicide intervention movement and the rest of society, which is to prevent it wherever possible*."[92] Faye Girsh, executive director of the Hemlock Society USA, emphasizes: "What we have been advocating for 17 years is legal aid in dying with the help of a physician."[93] She proposes that "In the case of a minor or an incompetent adult . . . some provision should be made [to terminate lives that] in the belief of the patient *or his agent are too burdensome to continue*."[94]

The Hemlock Society, together with the American Civil Liberties Union, had also filed an *amicus curiae* brief with the Supreme Court to support the right to PAS. They stated: "The right to doctor-assisted suicide applies just as well to deaths that are not self-administered—to individuals who are no longer mentally competent and to patients not terminally ill.... [The right] cannot stop short of a right to lethal injection or other forms of active killing."[95] The names "Hemlock Society" and "American Civil Liberties Union" are two more misnomers in the lexicon of "suicide assistance."

Anticipating the Supreme Court's decision in the case of *Compassion in Dying v. State of Washington*, a panel of prominent philosophers—including Thomas Nagel, Robert Nozick, John Rawls, Thomas Scanlon, Judith Jarvis Thomson, and headed by Ronald Dworkin, professor of jurisprudence at Oxford University and professor of law and philosophy at New York University—issued an appeal supporting the right to such assistance. The statement, written for the panel by Ronald Dworkin, begins with a powerful endorsement of CPSP: "[The panel recognizes] that people may make such momentous decisions impulsively or out of emotional depression.... States have a constitutionally legitimate interest in protecting individuals from irrational ... unstable decisions to hasten their own death."[96]

The philosophers emphasize their opposition to "*forcing* a competent dying patient to live in agony a few weeks longer,"[97] and say they are unable to discern significant differences between refusing treatment and receiving PAS, and praise PAS as a boon especially for poor people: "The most important benefit of legalized assisted suicide for poor patients however, might be better care while they live."[98] While this sounds uplifting, evidence from the Netherlands suggests that PAS and VE function, in fact, as substitutes for medical care for the terminally ill, not as incentives for improving such care. Brian Eads, a writer for *Reader's Digest*, reports: "In Holland, the key alternative to euthanasia—palliative care—is largely unavailable."[99]

The philosophers' brief concludes: "[D]eclaring that terminally ill patients in great pain do not have a constitutional right to control their own deaths, even in principle, seems alien to our constitutional system.... It would also undermine a variety of the Court's own past decisions, including the carefully constructed position on abortion."[100] This argument rests on the analogy between abortion and physician-assisted suicide, which is inappropriate and misleading, as I showed earlier in this chapter. After the Supreme Court unanimously rejected the claim that the Constitution guarantees a right to PAS,[101] Dworkin published a rebuttal titled, "Assisted Suicide: What the Court Really Said."[102] The title implies that we cannot understand what the Court said by reading what the Justices wrote, unless Dworkin explains what they "really said." The decision, Dworkin declares, is "deceptive.... [Justice] Stevens's opinion, though technically a vote against those who challenged the prohibitory statutes, was in fact *a vote for all they asked*."[103] Obviously that is not true. If it were, Justice Stevens would have voted to affirm the right to PAS. What the Supreme Court "really said" was, *inter alia*, that PAS was not a matter for the *federal (national) government* to decide.

Dworkin does not help his case by defending the practice of Dutch doctors who kill infants to make their parents more comfortable (by relieving the burden of care for the children). He writes: "The [Dutch] cases described as euthanasia 'without a patient's request' . . . included, for example . . . cases of just-born infants who would have died within days anyway." Doctors are fallible. Sometimes they predict that an infant is doomed, yet he survives and becomes a healthy, productive person. This does not concern Dworkin. He wants to relieve the parents' suffering. He continues: "and whose prompt death, at their parents' request, saved those parents agony." That is the rationalization that launched the Nazi euthanasia program.

Clearly, persons who look to the Law to support medical killing—call it what they may—find justification for them in the Constitution; persons who look to Religion for such support, find justification in divine revelation; and persons who look to Medicine for such support, find justification in emergency treatment. They all labor in the same garden whose poisonous fruit hardens the heart of Authority with compassion to kill. I feel compelled to repeat, and repeat once again, that giving Authority—in this case, physicians—more authority over how we die does not increase our autonomy. Authorities—priests, politicians, and physicians—have always had the power to kill and have exercised that power when it suited their purposes. What the Authorities abhor is letting people kill themselves, correctly recognizing in that act the individual's revolt against authority and his assertion of autonomy.

THE PERILS OF A "RIGHT" TO SUICIDE AS A "RIGHT" TO TREATMENT

Social policies that discourage people from assuming responsibility for their behavior encourage politicians to draft more legislation to protect people from their lack of responsibility for themselves, generating a vicious cycle of granting more power to bureaucrats, thereby further undermining the liberty and responsibility of the people.

The psychiatric reformers' struggle to guarantee mental patients a "right to treatment" became, in practice, the psychiatrists' right to treat patients against their will.[104] The marijuana reformers' fight to medicalize the use of cannabis has spawned more fanatical antidrug laws.[105] The assisted-suicide reformers' efforts to medicalize suicide are destined to be similarly counterproductive, threatening to transform the right to PAS into the physicians' right to kill patients by giving them this "treatment." There is evidence for this assumption.

In October 1997, the Supreme Court upheld the 1994 Oregon Death with Dignity Act.[106] In March 1998, Oregon's Health Services Commission added, for Medicaid patients, "doctor-assisted suicide to other forms of 'comfort care' for any 'terminal illness, regardless of diagnosis.' " Dr. Alan Bates, the head of the commission, explained: "Can we say to the people of Oregon this is something everyone else can have, but you [the poor] cannot? . . . If dying people with private insurance can pay for medical help in taking their own lives, why should poor people be deprived of the same opportunity? Anything less would be discriminatory."[107] The federal government did not take these attacks on its war on drugs lying down. In April, without waiting for the Supreme Court to issue its ruling about PAS, the U.S. Senate "passed a bill that bars Medicare and Medicaid payments for assisted suicide . . . [and authorized appropriating] funds for *suicide prevention programs* among the terminally ill."[108]

In an important earlier federal riposte against the DWDA (in November 1997), Thomas Constantine, the administrator of the Drug Enforcement Administration (DEA, an agency of the Justice Department), correctly noted that prescribing drugs for suicide "was not a legitimate medical use under the federal drug laws . . . [and] warned that the government would impose severe sanctions on any doctor who writes a prescription for lethal doses of medicine for a patient."[109] Six months later, Constantine was rebuffed by his boss. In June 1998, Attorney General Janet Reno promised "that doctors who use the law to prescribe lethal drugs to terminally-ill patients will not be prosecuted . . . there was no evidence that Congress meant for the DEA to have the novel role of resolving the profound moral and ethical questions involved in the issue [PAS]." Evidence to the contrary notwithstanding, Reno maintained that "the drug laws were intended to block illegal trafficking in drugs and did not cover situations like the Oregon suicide law."[110] Reno's assertion that the drug laws were not intended to cover "situations like the Oregon suicide law" is true: When the drug laws were enacted, there were no "suicide laws." However, her assertion is, as a practical matter, false: if it were true, physicians would not realistically fear prosecution for "overprescribing" narcotics for patients with chronic pain.

Orrin Hatch (R-Utah), chairman of the Senate Judiciary Committee, immediately protested that Reno "had misunderstood the federal drug laws." Representative Chris Smith (R-NJ) added that he "is confident that there will be a legislative attempt to undo Reno's ruling."[111] By September the House was considering a bill that "would allow the Federal Drug Enforcement Administration to investigate and punish any physician who prescribes lethal doses of drugs with the intent of assisting in a patient's suicide."[112]

The foregoing actions demonstrate that American laws regulating drug use and suicide have become increasingly capricious and contradictory and are apt to reverse course at a moment's notice. These features characterize the legal systems of despotic governments. In our headlong embrace of the Therapeutic State, we are creating a society at once anarchic and tyrannical, regulated by a mindless combination of illegal lawfulness and legal lawlessness; in short, a polity that makes a mockery of the Rule of Law.

6

Perverting Suicide
Killing as Treatment

The nationwide policy of administering euthanasia to mentally defective people, psychotics, epileptics . . . was in violation of the [National Socialist] penal code. . . . The program was regulated according to the motto: "The needle belongs in the hand of the doctor."

—German euthanasia policy, 1938–1945[1]

Anyone who takes the life of another on that person's express and serious request will be punished with a prison sentence of a maximum of twelve years. . . . [A] physician will be judged guilty but not culpable if he or she performs euthanasia or assists suicide in the correct way. *This legal decision is based on the concept of the state of emergency within which the physician acts.*

—Dutch euthanasia policy today[2]

If acts of euthanasia could be carried out only by a member of the medical profession, with the concurrence of a second doctor, it is not likely that the propensity to kill would spread unchecked throughout the community.

—Peter Singer (1993)[3]

Political freedom, as that idea has been understood in the English-speaking world, rests largely on the rule of law, which the foremost nineteenth-century English constitutional scholar Albert Venn Dicey (1835–1922) defined as "the equality of all citizens before the law; the unacceptableness of *raison d'etat* [reason of state] as an excuse for an unlawful act; and the observance of the old maxim, *nullum crimen sine lege* [no crime without law]."[4] The opposite of the Rule of Law is not lawlessness but arbitrariness, that is, laws capriciously interpreted, unpredictably enforced, and freely transgressed by superiors in dealing with subordinates. In addition to the Rule of Law, political freedom requires respect for private property, the strict enforceability of contracts, and a government whose powers are limited by a constitution.

- In the Constitutional State, relations between agents of the State and citizens are regulated by the Rule of Law: Acts not prohibited by the criminal law are legal (not punished by the State), whereas acts prohibited by the criminal law are illegal (punished by the State).

- In the Therapeutic State, relations between agents of the State and citizens are regulated by the Rule of Therapeutic Discretion: Some acts not prohibited by the criminal law (for example, "hearing voices" and attempted suicide) are sometimes *de facto* illegal, punished by sanctions called "therapeutic"; whereas some acts prohibited by the criminal law (for example, euthanasia in the Netherlands, prescribing controlled substances for suicide in the United States), are *de facto* legal for some people, authorized by the government and practiced by professionals.

With increasing momentum, the American people and the American government are embracing the principle that certain acts prohibited by law ought to be permitted if prescribed by physicians for persons identified as "patients."[5] The policy of authorizing the medical use of (otherwise illegal) marijuana is an example. Federal law prohibits the use of marijuana. California law prohibits growing marijuana but permits its medical use. How does the State obtain marijuana intended for medical use? By distributing marijuana confiscated under its criminal statutes. The policy of authorizing the medical use of (otherwise illegal) assistance with suicide would greatly expand this pernicious principle and the practices based on it. The medical and media campaigns rationalizing these practices as therapeutic procedures are driving the last nail into the coffin of the free society understood as the Constitutional State.

PHYSICIAN-ASSISTED SUICIDE AND EUTHANASIA IN THE NETHERLANDS

The principal parties concerned with medical care—and contending for its control—are the patient, the doctor, and the State. If medical care is primarily a private affair (a service traded in the market), then access to medical services is controlled largely by patients, and if it is primarily a public affair (a tax-paid service the State owes its citizens), then access to medical services is controlled largely by the State. Properly speaking, State-controlled medicine—which begins with medical licensure and ends with the physician as government employee and the patient as recipient of a government service—ought to be called "socialist medicine."*

That capitalism and socialism—the private versus the public ownership of goods and services—are in conflict is stating a truism. However, whenever we consider how people gain access to medical goods and services (drugs and physicians), it is necessary to keep this truism in mind, lest we forget that State regulation of medical goods and services is a species of State regulation and hence a political matter.

Medical Killing in the Netherlands: Opinions and Practices

The term "physician-assisted suicide" (PAS) refers to a physician writing a prescription for a patient, typically for a lethal amount of barbiturates, which the patient ingests in the physician's absence when and if he chooses to do so. The term "voluntary euthanasia" (VE) refers to a physician putting a patient to sleep, not for the purpose of inducing anesthesia for surgery or otherwise relieving pain, but for the purpose of causing death by injecting a lethal drug. Two points need to be emphasized at the outset. One is that although it is widely believed that in the Netherlands PAS is legal, it is not. The other is that euthanasia is more prevalent than assisted suicide and that "the Dutch make little moral or legal distinction between the two."[6]

Reports about the scope of euthanasia in the Netherlands vary. In 1997, Pieter V. Admiraal, probably the world's leading spokesperson for the right to VE, estimated that each year about 2,500 Dutch citizens die by means of PAS, another 4,000 by "active euthanasia"; and that "in about 1,000 cases [per annum] . . . life was terminated *without the explicit request of the patient*."[7] According to a feature article in *Time* magazine, the figures (in 1997) were 3,600 cases of PAS and VE (undifferentiated), of which about 900 fell into the category of "termination of life without the request of the patient."[8]

Observers of euthanasia policy in the Netherlands agree that Dutch laws regulating euthanasia are observed in the breach and that physicians and the public prefer it that way. In a decision celebrating the grandeur of medical discretion, the Dutch High Court, contrary to its officially proclaimed principles, declared: "[U]nbearable *mental suffering can in exceptional cases justify physician-assisted suicide, even if there is no concurrent medical disease*, and that the degree of suffering rather than its cause is decisive."[9] Most Dutch psychiatrists agree that PAS and VE are acceptable options "for pa-

*Because the term "socialism" reasonates with National Socialism and International Socialism (Communism), and because the American health care system is, in fact, already largely statist, it is politically incorrect to call it "socialist." Describing the system as regulated by "market forces" or "market competition," although politically correct, is factually incorrect.

tients whose suffering is based on a *mental disorder* in the absence of terminal (or even physical) illness."[10] Note that American psychiatrists diagnose such patients as suffering "clinical depression" and use this diagnosis to justify hospitalizing and treating the patient against his will.

In a 1993 opinion poll, the Dutch people were asked: "Do you think that someone always has the right to have his life terminated when he is in an unacceptable position without any prospect?"* Seventy-eight percent of the respondents said yes; ten percent said no.[11] Note that the question makes no reference to illness, doctors, drugs, medicine, or suicide. Pollsters and those polled probably assumed that doctors would be doing the terminating.

Euthanasia enjoys the support of the Dutch Royal Society of Medicine, of respected medical and lay groups, and of the majority of the people. The Dutch Voluntary Euthanasia Society issues "Euthanasia Passports" to its members, enabling those who carry it to indicate their consent to the procedure. We are not told whether the society also issues "Anti-Euthanasia Passports," enabling persons to forgo this free medical benefit.

How do Dutch doctors justify and view their euthanasia program? They justify it the same way as do American advocates of PAS: They too believe that medical killing affirms the patient's autonomy. Admiraal writes: "In discussing voluntary euthanasia it must be borne in mind that this is not possible without also considering the right of autonomy. . . . The patient has the indisputable right . . . to request euthanasia."[12] Of course, everyone has a right to *request* anything; he has also a "right" to be disappointed. Clearly, what Admiraal means is that some people, by virtue of being "suffering patients," have an "entitlement-right" to being killed by a doctor. Actually, the only right a Dutch patient has with respect to VE is to assume the role of medical supplicant.

Bert Keizer, a Dutch physician working in a nursing home where VE is routinely practiced, offers a candid insider's look at euthanasia in the Netherlands. Deeply conscious of modern man's passion to evade the existential duty to give meaning to his life, he remarks: "We no longer know what we're doing here or why, so we have taken to looking at our molecules, find out what they're up to. . . . [W]e know more about sodium than about ourselves. . . . You can't ask what the use of life is, the way you can of a hammer: to drive in nails."[13] Free of illusions about depression as a disease, Keizer scoffs at the term "anti-depressant," which he aptly characterizes as "one of those pincer words with which we dare to pick up things we wouldn't otherwise touch. If you were to call such a pill 'anti-despairant,' then it would

---

*Prison inmates serving long sentences meet this criterion, yet much attention is devoted to preventing their suicide.

be clear what we're talking about *and* that such a pill does not exist."[14] He then presents this disheartening vignette:

Picture the tragedy: you're 82, alive and kicking, you manage on your own . . . and then disaster strikes: you wake up after a stroke. To say you're seriously impaired sounds like a joke. You can't pee or pass stool without help, you can't speak or stand up, or sit up even. . . . Now to avoid having to look at this misery, we say: Mr. A. is suffering from depression. . . . So he gets an anti-depressant, which is our way of drawing a curtain over that misery. For that stupid pill is for us, bystanders.[15]

If Keizer's account is true (and we have no reason to doubt it), patient autonomy in the Dutch euthanasia system is—to put it mildly—a cruel hoax. He details the story of a man waiting to receive the lethal cocktail he has been promised. Frustrated by what seems to him an incomprehensible delay, the dying man threatens to set fire to the curtains in his room if his request is denied. He sets the fire and is punished for it. Keizer writes:

After this incident, they packed him off to psychiatry. . . . I pass him in the corridor where he sits. . . . He calls out to me from afar, "Doctor, doctor, when are you going to give me euthanasia?" I admonish him, "Please, not in this way. Think about the other patients." Later, in his room, I ask him: "Do you understand that you can't just call out for euthanasia as if it's an aspirin." "No," he says drily. What do I do with this clown?[16]

The physician cannot honor the patient's direct request for PAS/VE. If he did, it would unmask the procedure as a medical ritual, not a *bona fide treatment*.* Instead, the patient must pretend that he will receive his last medical rites (the lethal drug) when his physician decides that he, the patient, is "medically ready" for it. It is this pathetic humiliation of dying people, with nothing to look forward to but dying at their doctor's hands, that supporters of PAS call "respecting patient autonomy." Keizer soberly concludes:

The cruel thing about old age, especially extreme old age, is that it is like a trap that you wander into completely unawares. When you want to turn round to dash to the exit, the trap has snapped shut, without your noticing. There is no answer to the question: when should you end your life? Ten minutes before the fatal stroke which

---

*Similarly, the American psychiatrist cannot honor the patient's direct request for admission to a mental hospital. If he did, it would unmask civil commitment as a medical ritual, not a *bona fide treatment*. Instead, the patient must pretend that he will be admitted when his psychiatrist decides that he, the patient, "requires" hospitalization because he is "dangerous to himself or others." In other words, the patient's request for admission to the mental hospital must be concealed: He must "commit" schizophrenia or a "bizarre" crime to achieve his goal.

is going to maim you mentally beyond recognition, or a year before you are so demented that you don't know any more what it is you would end.[17]

Keizer's account documents that physicians practicing euthanasia in the Netherlands routinely deny direct requests for euthanasia and are proud of it; in short, it is they, not the patients, who decide who dies and when he dies. A case cited by Jay Branegan, the Amsterdam correspondent for *Time* magazine, is illustrative. The patient is afflicted with multiple sclerosis but is not terminally ill. His repeated requests for euthanasia are denied. After some months pass, the physician contacts *the patient's wife* and informs her that he "is ready for it." The patient comes home from the nursing home and the doctor "administers the poison." Afterward, his wife says: "I'm convinced we did the right thing."[18] That, I think, is the point: convincing patients, families, physicians, and the public that when the physician "administers the poison," he and everyone else are doing "the right thing." That makes the Dutch practice of euthanasia "normal" and hence "ethical."

How do Dutch doctors know when the patient is ready for VE? Herbert Hendin's report about his experiences with VE in the Netherlands may be part of the answer. He writes: "Euthanasia is becoming much more of a habit and routine. I even had one hospital doctor complaining to me that a colleague had killed one of his patients because he needed a bed."[19]

Although Keizer is dissatisfied with the way VE is practiced in the Netherlands, he seems unaware that the practice is intrinsically flawed, both morally and politically. Providing medical services entails costs, whether paid by the patient out of his own funds, by his private insurance policy, or by the government from its tax receipts. The economic incentives of patient and society coincide if the patient opts for VE, but diverge if he opts for expensive medical care. Two American critics of PAS point out that "Doing less or withholding treatment can certainly decrease costs. . . . In terms of cost effectiveness alone, few procedures would be ranked higher than assisted suicide."[20] Instead of confronting the moral and political-economic problems posed by VE (in a system of "free" medical care), Keizer hopes to *humanize* the technique. He writes: "There was or is no ritual for euthanasia the way we know it, because this is a rare occurrence in history. I believe there is a stronger call now for ritual, because we have to deal with a more accurate prognosis."[21] What Keizer and his colleagues are doing is, indeed, novel, because the Therapeutic State is novel. His recommendation, however, is naive. What we need is not a new ritual for bureaucratized medical killing, but the rejection of legally and medically formalized schemes of mercy killing by doctors, accompanied by a critical attitude toward the deceptions and self-deceptions intrinsic to policies regulating PAS and VE.

"Gedogen": Hypocrisy as a Virtue

In April 1997, Gerrit van der Wal, a professor of social medicine at Amsterdam's Free University, granted an interview to syndicated columnist Ellen Goodman. Goodman wanted to know how the Dutch people reconcile the legal prohibition of PAS and VE with the flourishing practice of these procedures. The answer, van der Wal explained to Goodman, lies in the Dutch word, *"gedogen,"* which the dictionary translates as "tolerance": "If the word is not easily translated, perhaps it is because the concept is so Dutch. *Gedogen* describes a formal condition somewhere between forbidden and permitted. Here drugs are *gedogen*. They remain illegal, but soft drugs like marijuana and hashish are available in duly licensed coffee shops that dot this city. And here, too, euthanasia is *gedogen*."[22] In other words, the Dutch people approve of a medical-legal system in which "the ending of a life by a doctor remains illegal, but doctors who follow careful guidelines may grant their patients' death wishes";[23] or, as Admiraal puts it: "Legally euthanasia should remain a crime, but if a physician... shortens the life of the patient... the court will have to judge whether there was a conflict of duties which could justify the act of the physician."[24]

It does not follow, however, that attributing the acceptance of involuntary euthanasia to *gedogen* and treating *gedogen* as if it were *ipso facto* praiseworthy makes involuntary euthanasia (or PAS or VE, for that matter) praiseworthy as well. If the end is unacceptable, acceptable means cannot justify it. Moreover, in this case, the means are also unacceptable. I for one am revolted by a legal system that simultaneously prohibits *and* licenses the sale of a particular good or service.

Goodman, like other critics of Dutch euthanasia practices, deplores that Dutch physicians regularly euthanize patients who do not meet the criteria for receiving such "assistance" and that "most euthanasia deaths are still (and illegally) *not reported to the government.*"[25] As if it were a defense against this charge, Dutch euthanasia experts tell Americans that their system is not for export and give this reason for it: "The difference between Holland and America is universal health care. No one here chooses to die to protect their family finances."[26] Evidently, the Dutch people find it comforting that patients killed by doctors do not have to pay for the service and that the doctors get no fee for it. They consider this arrangement a protection against "abuses." I consider it evidence for the wisdom of the adage, "He who pays the piper, calls the tune." Only a political naif or a socialist fanatic could believe that finances influence health care only in a capitalist system.

The moral dilemmas intrinsic to the physician-patient relationship are grave enough when the patient is a competent adult. When the patient is a mental patient (presumed to be incompetent) or a child, the dilemmas are even graver. Normally, the child's parent or legal guardian represents and protects his best medical interests: He is legally authorized to give or refuse consent to diagnostic and therapeutic procedures performed on the child. When, for whatever reason, this protection is lacking, we are on the brink of a moral abyss: Who shall protect the child? I raise the question not to answer it (I do not know how to do that), but to place the practice of euthanizing children—which evidently is gaining popularity in the Netherlands—in its proper context.

Nat Hentoff, a writer with impeccable credentials as a civil libertarian, reports that Dutch parents of disabled children are often rebuked with "statements such as 'What? Is that child still alive? How can one love such a child? . . . Such a thing should be given an injection.' . . . There seems to be little tolerance for disabled children and the parents who raise them."[27] Clearly, universal health care in the Netherlands has not made life more secure for handicapped children or crippled old people. "A 1995 study . . . disclosed that 23 percent of the doctors interviewed reported that they had euthanized a patient without his or her explicit request. . . . At least half of the Dutch physicians involved . . . suggested euthanasia to the patient."[28]

Hentoff cites Richard Fenigsen, a Dutch cardiologist and critic of VE, as his source for the following case of a three-year-old boy who "had spina bifida but was otherwise in fair general condition. For two days he did not feel quite well and his parents asked for euthanasia." A nurse who opposed the decision and her husband offered to adopt the child. The offer was turned down and "the nurse was reprimanded because by involving her husband in the adoption offer she violated professional confidentiality. . . . The boy was killed by physicians with drugs administered with intravenous drip."[29]

By citing only critics of the Dutch euthanasia policy, I do not want to create the impression that it has no supporters—in the United States or elsewhere. The opposite is the case. One of the famous champions of that system is the well-known philosopher-ethicist and animal rights activist Peter Singer. His not-so-hidden agenda—which he shares with most supporters of medical killings of all sorts—is waging a propaganda campaign against individualism and capitalism, and for medical statism (the Therapeutic State). After praising the Dutch system of medical killing, Singer remarks: "Americans, in particular, would do well to remember that the Netherlands is a welfare state that provides a high standard of health care and social security to all its citizens. No patients need to ask for euthanasia because they are unable to afford good health care."[30] The last sentence implies that Americans *need to ask for euthanasia because they are unable to afford good health care.* The fact that no one in America asks his physician to kill him because he cannot afford medical care does not prevent Singer from making such an assertion and does not stop many people from believing such rubbish. Not surprisingly, Singer is also enthusiastic about *gedogen* (although he does not use the word), specifically about the fact that "Although the [Dutch] parliament did not repeal the law that makes mercy killing a criminal offence," such killing is widely practiced.[31] Indeed, Singer predicts that "the citizens of several other countries will join the Dutch in finding a way to gain control of how they die."[32] This is an unconscionable misstatement of the facts. As we have seen, Dutch citizens have not found "a way to gain control of how they die"; they have only found a way to gain control—if one can call it "control"—of how they can ask doctors to let them die, on the doctors' terms. Nevertheless, Singer believes he is supporting patient autonomy.

In sum, the desire to medically legitimize medical killing has led the Dutch people and their government to collude in a gigantic charade: Dutch criminal law prohibits PAS/VE; the Dutch law enforcement system treats practicing PAS/VE as a noncrime; Dutch physicians systematically violate the laws and guidelines regulating PAS/VE and for doing so are admired as compassionate professionals, uncorrupted by fee-for-service incentives. Dutch physicians and the Dutch public alike embrace the inversion of the rule of law into the rule of therapeutic discretion as a morally exalted form of illegality ("*gedogen*"); the Dutch people are considered law-abiding lovers of liberty; and the Netherlands is looked upon as a model liberal society.

THE HOLOCAUST: PHYSICIAN-ASSISTED MURDER

We cannot understand medicine under National Socialism unless we recognize that the practices *we* call "medical atrocities" were the inevitable results of the German people's effort to *use medicine as an instrument of the state to protect them from persons they regarded as their enemies and whom they defined as "sick."* The National Socialist euthanasia program did not arise in a historical vacuum. It arose from and expressed the ideals of *eugenics* as a biological doctrine of race-improvement and was based on and implemented the principles of *socialist medicine* as a political system willing to sacrifice the individual for the benefit of the collective.

The notion of racial hygiene and its master metaphors of waging war against a horde of dangerous parasites—criminals, homosexuals, the insane, and other "defectives"—is an integral part of eugenics-as-euthanasia and of public health as politics.[33] The principle of racial hygiene, the emblem of the corruption of biological science in the service of the state,[34] was built upon internationally shared eugenic concepts and images that flourished in the West long before it became genocidal State policy in National Socialist Germany. Its rhetorical apparatus—typified by the declaration of Gerhard Wagner, head of the National Socialist Physicians' League, that

"Jews were a 'diseased race' and Judaism was 'disease incarnate' "[35]—was developed and popularized during the years preceding World War I. Martin S. Pernick, professor of history at the University of Michigan, correctly observes: "Almost no one today remembers that Americans ever died in the name of eugenics, much less that such deaths were highly publicized and widely supported. . . . Both eugenics and euthanasia provided assessments of which lives were not worth living. 'Eugenics' could mean deciding who was 'better-not-born,' and 'euthanasia' could mean deciding who was 'better-off-dead.' "[36]

One self-proclaimed American socialist predicted that "the day of the parasite [he was referring to capitalists as well as to defectives], who eats his bread without earning it, will soon pass." Others warned that "Our streets are infested with an Army of the Unfit—a dangerous, vicious army of death and dread."[37] The unfit, Pernick emphasizes, "did not simply *have* a disease; they *were* the disease."[38] Experts taught the public to understand that "to kill off the weakling born [is] nature's way"; that "death is the great and lasting disinfectant"; and that "in prolonging the lives of defectives we are tampering with the functioning of the social kidneys."

Interest in eugenics-as-euthanasia was rekindled in Germany after World War I. The argument that the destruction of "lives not worth living" is a humane medical act, serving the best interests of both the euthanized person (patient) and the society he burdens (the State), in part reflected the economic and political demoralization of the German public in the aftermath of the war. In 1920, a group of German parents with handicapped children were asked whether they would want their children put to death. Seventy-three percent said yes and expressed "the hope that they would never be told the true cause of their child's death."[39]

Initially, the class of persons considered living "lives not worth living" was limited to severely handicapped children and hopelessly ill adults. Under National Socialism, mental patients, Jews, Gypsies, and homosexuals were added to the list. The world-famous biologist Johann von Uexkull maintained that members of "alien races . . . [are] parasites."[40] The idea that persons who were assigned to these statuses were *enemies of society* who deserved to be destroyed was, as I noted, not limited to German physicians and scientists. In 1935, Alexis Carrel, the French-American inventor of the iron lung and a Nobel Prize winner in medicine, declared: "The criminal and the insane should be humanely and economically disposed of in small euthanasia institutions supplied with proper gases."[41] In 1941, Foster Kennedy, one of America's leading psychiatrists, declared: "I am in favor of euthanasia for those hopeless ones who should never have been born. . . . I believe it is a merciful and kindly thing to relieve that defective of the agony of living."[42]

The Socialist Foundations of the Medical Holocaust

The socialist foundations of German medicine were laid down by Chancellor Otto von Bismarck's (1815–1898) pioneering social security programs. As a result, medicine became a partly private and partly public enterprise, in which the physician played the double role of medical practitioner *and* medical bureaucrat.[43]

After World War I, the German Association of Socialist Physicians lent fresh impetus to turning medicine into an arm of the State. The association's motto was: "Every doctor who wishes to practice his art effectively must be a socialist." The president and cofounder of the association, Ernst Simmel—a psychiatrist-psychoanalyst and close associate of Freud's —called capitalism "the greatest malady affecting industrial society" and demanded the "socialization of health care."[44] The association's program extended far beyond the then-normal bounds of medicine, to social policies such as improving housing and nutrition for poor people and the right to abortion.[45]

After Hitler's ascension to power, the German Association of Socialist Physicians was declared illegal. Most of its Jewish members emigrated. Proctor cogently notes that "in a number of areas the concerns of socialist physicians overlapped with those of the Nazis. . . . Both advocated an increased role of the state in the administration of public health and viewed the task of medicine as fundamentally a political one";[46] and that "some of Germany's most influential advocates of social hygiene . . . defended a qualified form of racial hygiene."[47]

The exemplar of the defenseless patient whose life others may consider "not worth living" is the child deemed defective. The desire of parents to rid themselves of such children was an important initial impetus for what became the Holocaust. In 1938, the father of a child born blind, retarded, and without an arm or a leg, wrote to Hitler asking him to grant the child " 'mercy death' or euthanasia."[48] Within a year, the policy for the medical mass murder of human beings was formalized: The National Socialist Party's Committee for the Scientific Treatment of Severe, Genetically Determined Illnesses issued an order requiring physicians and midwives to register with the health authorities any child born with "idiocy . . . microcephaly or hydrocephaly of a progressive and severe nature; deformities of any kind, especially missing limbs, malformations of the head, or spina bifida [etc.]." Such children were sent to *psychiatric institutions* for the explicit purpose of being killed with morphine or cyanide or by starvation. Two years later, the age limit for the children's euthanasia program was raised to include youths up to seventeen years old.[49]

Among the victims of the child-psychiatric holocaust were many physically healthy youngsters who were sent to mental hospitals for trivial problems by parents gulled by psychiatric propaganda. One of the most sickening episodes of this horror story took place in Vienna, where, "In Doctor [Heinrich] Gross's children's hospital, you stuttered, you died; you had a harelip, you died; you wet the bed, you died." Despite repeated exposures after the war and a mountain of evidence against him, the Austrian government has heaped honors on Gross.[50]

The German people supported the medical killing of "defective children": "Many parents wrote to hospitals to ask if their child could be relieved of his or her misery and be granted euthanasia." It is a testament to the power of ideas that Jewish children were initially *excluded* from this operation, "on the ground that they did not deserve the 'merciful act' (*Wohltat*)* of euthanasia. . . . *Jews were explicitly declared not to deserve euthanasia.*"[51] Only in 1941 were Jewish mental patients ordered to be killed, "not because they met the criteria required for medical killing (euthanasia), but because they were Jews."[52]

Pari passu, Germany's leading anthropologists and psychiatrists met, in 1938, to plan the systematic killing of *mental patients:* "They all agreed that *a law which permitted the killing of psychiatric patients was necessary.*" Having decided that, they deliberated about how to justify and what to call such killing: Some of the experts suggested calling it "granting of medical assistance to die"; others proposed phrases such as "law for the granting of last aid" and "law for the granting of special or specially assisted help."[53] Austrian psychiatrists called the mass murder of "handicapped and 'anti-social' [*sic*]" children "death accelerations."[54] The idea of granting mercy death to "defective" children struck a responsive chord among German artists and writers, who joined doctors demanding that the State give physicians permission to "grant mercy death" to patients who would be better off dead. German advocates of mercy killing in the 1930s, like American advocates of physician-assisted suicide today, systematically conflated and confused self-killing (suicide) with medical killing rationalized as compassion for the "suffering patient" and with medical killing rationalized as compassion for an "overburdened society."

The basic rationale that supported medical killing in Nazi Germany was the conviction, *based on a deeply "idealistic" belief in socialism,* that defending the nation against persons diagnosed as "parasites" requires abolishing the very idea of private health as distinct from public health. In the National Socialist state, health was synonymous with public health; everything related to health was, *ipso facto,* a matter of legitimate State control. In this respect, Nazi Germany was a particular version of the Therapeutic State.

---

*Literally, *wohl* is "well." The term implies health or enjoyment; a more precise, albeit awkward, translation of *Wohltat* would be "well-deed."

Although Proctor draws no parallels between the treatment of mental patients in Nazi Germany and in the West, he notes that physicians pathologized not only Jews but also "Gypsies, communists, homosexuals ... and a wide class of 'antisocials' (alcoholics, prostitutes, drug addicts, the homeless, and other groups) [all of whom] were marked for destruction."[55]

Killing as Psychiatric Treatment

Ever since the early work on intelligence testing, the concepts of mental hygiene and racial hygiene were closely connected.[56] Thus, it was easy to progress from removing a person from society because he fails to meet criteria of racial hygiene to removing him because he fails to meet criteria of mental hygiene. According to the postwar testimony of Hitler's personal physician, Karl Brandt, "Hitler decided, even before he became Reich Chancellor in 1933, that he would one day try to eliminate the mentally ill."[57] This seemingly bizarre idea is, in fact, a logical extension of the traditional psychiatric view that the chronic mental patient is a nonperson (a person without rights or obligations) and a monstrous extension of the "time-honored" psychiatric practice of expelling such persons from society.[58]

In 1939, German psychiatrists began the systematic extermination of mental patients. It is now widely believed that this program was legal—that is, in conformity with Nazi laws. It was not: Like the prohibition of VE in the Netherlands today, "The nationwide policy of administering euthanasia to mentally defective people, psychotics, epileptics ... was in violation of the national penal code."[59] The prohibition of medical killing in Nazi Germany helped neither the patients selected for murder nor the doctors reluctant to act as executioners: "[Physicians] who were unable to flee into the army to remove themselves from this conflict of duties found themselves facing 'elimination.' "[60]

Grotesquely, the Nazi physicians were eager to prevent the "abuses" of the euthanasia program, by which they meant the practice of "therapeutic mercy killing" by nonmedical personnel. Karl Brandt stressed that "gassing should only be done by physicians." The program was regulated "according to the motto: 'The needle belongs in the hand of the doctor.' "[61] Between 1939 and 1941, more than 70,000 patients in German mental hospitals had been gassed and cremated. The decision about who deserved euthanasia was "made by psychiatric consultants, most of whom were professors in key universities."[62]

The longer the medical killings went on, the more intensely the Nazi hierarchy seemed to believe its own propaganda that it was a *medical* activity. In 1943 Himmler issued a decree "that only physicians trained in anthropology should carry out selection for killing, and supervise the killings themselves, in extermination camps."[63] Benno Muller-Hill, professor of genetics at the University of Cologne, remarks: "The psychiatrists recommended 'forced-labor therapy' for patients who had by some accident survived the euthanasia programme.... Auschwitz resembled the psychiatric institutions for extermination in that physicians were in charge of the 'selection' and killing. They had won these rights and were unwilling to have them taken away by others."[64] They need not have worried; the Nazi government had no intention of depriving them of their privileges.[65] As official doctrine had it, "doctors were never *ordered* to murder psychiatric patients and handicapped children. They were *empowered* to do so and fulfilled their task without protest, often on their own initiative."[66]

The history of medical killing in National Socialist Germany illustrates dramatically that once physicians agree to do the dirty work of society, that work becomes defined as standard medical practice, and physicians soon find themselves compelled to perform it or suffer the consequences of being branded as "unwilling to accept their medical responsibilities." (The penalties may range from loss of reputation to loss of career to loss of life.) American advocates of PAS now seek similar empowerment and promise that legalizing the act will not entail having to participate in the practice. The history of psychiatry suggests otherwise.

MEDICAL ETHICS AND THE STATE

Physicians occupy a unique role in society: We delegate control over our bodies and hence our lives to them and to them only. The relationship between physician and patient—comparable to that between parent and child, to which it is often compared—is, intrinsically, a relationship between a superior and a subordinate. Thus, it entails an actual or potential imbalance of power and the dangers associated with such an imbalance. The more the patient needs the physician's services, the weaker is his position in the relationship and the more he needs protection from the physician's abuse of his power. Who shall guard the medical guardians?

People have grappled with this problem since ancient times and have developed certain moral codes and legal rules to cope with it. One of the oldest such codes is the Hippocratic Oath prohibiting, among other things, physicians as physicians from killing. I believe we ought to view this rule not merely as a prudent prohibition but as a kind of medical taboo, similar to the incest taboo, that is, a rule beyond the purview of legislators and judges: *They themselves cannot repeal the prohibition.* I shall return to this point presently.

The second ancient safeguard against the abuse of medical power is the Roman medical maxim: *Primum non nocere!* (First, do no harm!). The physician must employ only such measures in his treatment of the patient that he believes will, on balance, benefit the patient. This rule is considered one of the commandments of modern medical ethics.

The third safeguard against the abuse of medical power is *consent*, that is, making the legitimacy of the physician's relationship to the patient contingent on the patient's permission for performing certain procedures on him (a permission the patient can at any time rescind). This principle, powerfully supported in modern English and American law, is often considered the first commandment of contemporary medical ethics.

Finally, we arrive at the fourth, and least appreciated, protection of the patient against the abuse of medical power: the market nexus, that is, the exchange of medical services, like other personal services, for money (an arrangement that presupposes two or more consenting parties). Although the market nexus provides important protections for the patient against medical dominance, it receives scant attention in the literature on bioethics. This is a vast subject not directly relevant to our subject. I shall briefly indicate the nature of these protections.

The relationship between sellers and buyers is never in perfect equilibrium. Sometimes there are more sellers than buyers, sometimes more buyers than sellers. For this and for other reasons, sometimes the sellers are more powerful, sometimes the buyers are. In the market nexus, if the patient is the buyer, if he is well informed about his medical needs and the available services, and if there are more physicians than the market can support, then the patient enjoys a large measure of protection from medical dominance and exploitation. Removing the medical relationship from the market destroys this safeguard. Receiving medical care *gratis*, as charity, or as a government-provided service, or even as a prepaid insurance benefit, renders the recipient-patient more dependent on and more subordinate to the physician than he would be if the physician were dependent on the patient for his income. In Medicine, he who pays the piper may not call the whole tune, nor should he, but he can always turn off the music. He who does not pay the medical piper *never* calls the therapeutic tune. This imbalance of power, intrinsic to socialist medicine, can never be corrected by giving people special "rights" as patients.

Beyond Consent: The Need for Absolute Limits on Medical Power

The proposition that it is immoral as well as illegal for a physician to perform a diagnostic or therapeutic intervention on a patient without the patient's consent is rarely, if ever, directly contested. However, although consent ought to be necessary for an act to qualify as a *medical intervention* it ought not be sufficient for it. Indeed, it is an established principle of medical ethics that there are certain acts from which the physician must abstain, regardless of whether the patient consents to the act (or even pleads for it): Killing the patient and having sexual relations with her (or him) are two such acts. These prohibitions are virtual taboos.

The life of primitive man is regulated largely by taboos, a type of prohibition for which modern man supposedly has no need. Regrettably, this not true. If it were, it would not have been so easy to turn physicians from healers into killers, most flagrantly in the service of the German, Japanese, and Soviet states, more subtly in the service of other modern states.

Whenever a group engages in evil—that is, whenever large numbers of people united in a cause commit acts that they would be unlikely to carry out alone—evil becomes defined as good. The medicalization of mass murder as a beneficial medical service is a terrifying example. Not by accident was the Holocaust prepared and preceded by the medicalized mass murder of mental patients. Years later, during the trial of Adolf Eichmann in Jerusalem, we were starkly reminded that, in our century, the physician as executioner debuted on the stage of history and that it would take time and effort to dislodge him from that role. In the course of defending Eichmann, his lawyer Robert Servatius blandly declared: "*Killing, too, is a medical matter.*"[67] Servatius did not say that killing *was* a medical matter. He said it *is* a medical matter. The evidence and arguments assembled in this book demonstrate that many people continue to believe that mercy killing and preventing persons from killing themselves are both medical matters.

The deformation of the German language that resurfaced during the Eichmann trial showed once again how easy it is to represent medical killing as a "therapeutic service." After the war, a physician who had worked in the Nazi death camps was asked: "How can you reconcile that [gassing of Jews] with your [Hippocratic] oath as a doctor?" He answered: "Of course I am a doctor and I want to preserve life. And out of respect for human life, I would remove the gangrenous appendix from a diseased body. The Jew is the gangrenous appendix in the body of mankind."[68]

The more we enlarge the categories we call "disease" and "treatment," the more we expand the scope of medicine and the power of the physician.[69] Narrowly defined, as it was by materialist physicians at the beginning of this century, the term "treatment" referred to the physician's effort to ameliorate or cure a bodily illness (with the consent of the patient). Broadly defined, as it is today, "treatment" includes abortion-as-contraception; killing some fetuses in utero to increase the chances of the remaining fetuses to survive; the use of drugs to increase stature or strength, to reduce weight, to satisfy the desire to be stimulated or tranquilized, and so forth. It is not surprising that many people regard PAS and VE also as "treatments." The authors of an essay in the *New England Journal of Medicine* write: "Physicians are logical candidates for participation [in PAS and VE].

They can assess a patient's medical and emotional status, and they know what pharmacological agents and modes of administration would meet the needs of particular patients . . . legislators will want to entrust the responsibility of assistance to physicians."[70]

Relaxing the unconditional prohibition against *legally authorized medical killing* (as PAS or VE) opens the floodgates to unlimited abuses of medical authority as power. If physician-assisted suicide is morally justified and legally permissible because the patient "needs" and requests it, and because we call it a "treatment," why should physician-assisted sex—or, indeed, *any consensual act* between physician and patient—not also be morally justified and legally permissible, provided we call it "treatment"? It follows that either the justification of PAS *as medical intervention* is untenable or that any act performed by a physician and rationalized as a treatment must *count as a bona fide "medical intervention"* and as such must be morally and legally acceptable.

Another reason why patient consent for a medical intervention ought not be a *sufficient* justification for it is that both custom and law treat consent as transferable, called the principle of substituted consent: Parents can give consent in lieu of their minor children, guardians in lieu of their incompetent wards, and, by extension, the State in lieu of its "childlike" citizens (the doctrine of *parens patriae*). This brings us back to the old dilemma, Who shall guard the guardians? Experience has shown how easy it is to transform the role of the physician from protector of the individual patient into the patient's persecutor in the service of the State. Psychiatry in particular has been, and continues to be, vulnerable to being turned into an instrument of State power.

There are many lessons the Holocaust can teach us. The lesson with which I want to conclude is that we ought to recognize that the aberrations of National Socialist medicine—which we ostensibly abhor—represent an exaggerated version of a type of conflict-resolution to which all modern states seeking "therapeutic" solutions for their moral-social problems are susceptible. The United States today meets that criterion to an alarming degree.

Rethinking Suicide

Death Control, the Final Responsibility

To every thing there is a season, and a time to every purpose under the heaven: A time to be born, and a time to die.
—Ecclesiastes, 3:1–2

Our ideas are reactions to a problem. If we do not live that problem, our concept of it, our interpretations of it, lack meaning and are in no way lively, full, living ideas.
—Jose Ortega y Gasset (1883–1955)[1]

Freedom granted only when it is known beforehand that its effects will be beneficial is not freedom. . . . Our faith in freedom does not rest on the foreseeable results in particular circumstances, but on the belief that it will, on balance, release more forces for the good than for the bad.
—Friedrich von Hayek (1889–1992)[2]

For more than two hundred years, the United States Supreme Court and lower courts have interpreted the Constitution. Their rulings range from affirming that we have a right to own other persons to denying that we have a right to own ourselves. This does not mean that we should ignore the Court's often wise counsel. It means that we ought to recognize that we draw on it as engaged polemicists, not as dispassionate scholars.

A "RIGHT TO SUICIDE"?

Some people say they want to kill themselves; some try and fail to kill themselves; some are merely suspected of wanting to kill themselves; and some explicitly deny that they want to kill themselves. Yet all of these persons are considered and called "suicidal." Declarations about wanting to commit suicide may be true or false. Attempts at suicide may be genuine (life-threatening) or bogus (not life-threatening). Yet both types of acts are considered and called "suicide attempts."

Should the State, by means of its criminal laws, punish persons called "suicidal"? In exercising its police power to maintain and promote "the healthful and sanitary condition of the general body of people or the community,"[3] should the State restrain such persons to protect the public? In exercising its duty as *parens patriae*, should the State restrain such persons by means of mental health laws aimed at protecting them from themselves? Or should the State leave them alone? As we have seen, persuasive arguments can be marshaled for all of these views. My aim, in this final chapter, is to argue that it ought to be morally and politically impermissible to use the coercive apparatus of the State to interfere with "suicidality." (The modern State does not interfere with suicide as an accomplished fact.) I begin therefore by citing some legal opinions that could, without stretching those writers' words, be interpreted as guaranteeing a "right to suicide," as a negative right. By this I mean that the government ought to be bound by law—the Constitution, if you like—to leave the citizen, *as* suicidal person, alone.

The difference between a positive right and a negative right is briefly this: A positive right is a claim on someone else's goods or services; in other words, it is a euphemism for an entitlement. Because the notion of a *right to suicide* (or physician-assisted suicide) entails an obligation by others to fulfill the reciprocal *duties* it entails, I reject the notion of a "right to suicide." However, I believe we have—and ought to be accorded—a "natural right" to be left alone to commit suicide. A truly humane society would recognize that option as a respected civil right. On more than one occasion, justices of the United States Supreme Court, as well as other judges, have, in effect, said just that.

The Right to Be Let Alone

"No right," declared the Court in 1891, "is held more sacred, or is more carefully guarded by the common law, than the right of every individual to possession and control of his own person, free from all restraint or interference of others. . . . The right to one's person may be said to be a right of complete immunity: to be let alone."[4]

In 1928, Supreme Court Justice Louis D. Brandeis (1856–1941) repeated that now-famous phrase and has since then been credited with it. He stated: "The makers of our Constitution sought to protect Americans in their beliefs, their thoughts, their emotions, and their sensations. They conferred, as against the Government, the right to be let alone—the most comprehensive of rights, and the right most valued by civilized men."[5]

It is difficult to reconcile these opinions with the practices of coercive suicide prevention, unless we assume that a diagnosis of mental illness automatically removes the diagnosed person from the class of human beings called "persons."[6] Moreover, in 1964, Chief Justice (then–Circuit Judge) Warren Burger wrote an opinion that can be interpreted only as meaning that mental patients, too, are entitled to the right to be let alone—to kill themselves. In an often-cited decision about the constitutionality of letting Jehovah's Witnesses reject life-saving blood transfusion, Burger repeated Brandeis's admonition and added: "Nothing in this utterance suggests that Justice Brandeis thought an individual possessed these rights only as to *sensible* beliefs, *valid* thoughts, *reasonable* emotions, or *well-founded* sensations. I suggest he intended to include a great many foolish, unreasonable, and even absurd ideas which do not conform, such as refusing medical treatment even at great risk."[7] Like the Jehovah's Witnesses who reject life-saving treatment for motives that are reasonable and right for them but unreasonable and wrong for others, suicidal persons reject coercive psychiatric suicide prevention (CPSP) for reasons that are right for them but wrong for others. If the former have a constitutional right to do so, why not also the latter?

A recent judicial ruling supports the view that the right to reject treatment is so similar to the right to be let alone to commit suicide as to make them medically, morally, and legally equivalent. In 1993, a prison physician in California sought a court order to permit him to use a surgical tube to feed and medicate a quadriplegic prisoner who had refused the intervention. The court ruled:

Right to refuse medical treatment is equally "basic and fundamental" and integral to concept of informed consent. Individual's right of personal autonomy to refuse medical treatment does not turn on wisdom, i.e., medical rationality . . . because health care decisions intrinsically concern one's subjective sense of well-being. . . . [T]the state has not embraced an unqualified or undifferentiated policy of preserving life at the expense of personal autonomy. . . . As a general proposition, the notion that the individual exists for the good of the state is, of course, quite antithetical to our fundamental thesis that the role of the state is to ensure a maximum of individual freedom of choice and conduct.[8]

Note that the physician proposed to treat the patient's decision to refuse food as if it were a *bona fide disease* (which it is not) and to tube feed a patient able to ingest food by mouth as if it were a *bona fide treatment* (which it is not). This decision has a direct and decisive bearing on the right to suicide: The court here granted the patient, as a matter of principle, the right to refuse treatment *irrationally*. This specification was long overdue. After all, the physician questions his patient's rationality *only* when the patient disagrees with him about the proposed treatment; this is a truism implicit in how the term "rational" is used in medical discourse. If an irrational prisoner has the right to be unmolested by physicians, on what ground would that right be denied an innocent person residing in his own home?

Asserting that we have a (negative) right to do something does not mean that exercising the right is morally meritorious. We have many rights—for example, to eat or drink to excess—whose exercise is decidedly not praiseworthy. The phrase *right to suicide* does not mean that suicide is desirable or that it is desirable that people commit suicide (for example, when they are fatally ill). It means only that agents of the State have no right or power to interfere, by prohibitions or punishments, with a person's decision to kill himself. Those who desire to prevent a particular person from committing suicide must be content with their power, such as it might be, to persuade him to change his mind. Freedom to decide matters that affect one's own health and the right to be let alone are both aspects of autonomy, a concept to which we must now turn.

THE ANATOMY OF AUTONOMY

The term "autonomy" is frequently misused and misunderstood, especially in contemporary writings about the physician-patient relationship. In part, this is because, since the end of World War II, the term "autonomy" underwent the same sort of metamorphosis as did the term "liberalism" after World War I. Prior to World War I, liberalism was the name of the political philosophy that regarded the State, possessing a monopoly on legal coercion, as a threat to individual liberty. In this vision, *protection from the State (liberty) is more important than protection by the State (security)*. Now called "classical liberalism" or "libertarianism," this view is now often erroneously attributed to statists called "conservatives."

Today, liberalism is the name of a political philosophy that regards the State as an organ of benevolence and compassion and therefore a source of protection and security for the individual. In this vision, *protection by the State (security) is more important than protection from State power (liberty)*. Called "liberalism" (sometimes capitalized), "communitarianism," "humanism," and "progressivism" by its adherents, it is called "socialism," "statism," and "totalitarianism" by its adversaries.

Clearly, we crave and need both liberty and security—a state strong enough to protect us from enemies within and without, yet restrained enough by constitutional guarantees and custom to respect personal liberty and responsibility. As individuals, we want to maximize our freedom, as persons-in-relation (e.g., husband-wife, doctor-patient), we want to maximize our security. These opposing human needs are reflected in the opposing moral principles and social policies usually identified as "guaranteeing human rights" and "protecting vulnerable persons." If we want to justify a person's *"right" to detach himself or herself from others* — for example, in the case of divorce or abortion—we appeal to his right to autonomy. On the other hand, if we want to justify a person's *"duty" to remain attached to others*—for example, in the case of caring for children or seriously ill patients—we appeal to his obligation to protect and provide for those who "naturally" depend on him. Instead of thinking carefully and critically about these conflicts and trying to resolve them by leaving people alone as much as possible to deal with them as they see fit, we deal with them collectively, coercively, and inconsistently, flipping from autonomy to paternalism and back again.

Autonomy: Its Meanings and Uses

Webster's Dictionary defines autonomy as "The quality or state of being independent, free, and self-directing." The term derives from the Greek root *auto*, meaning self, and *nomos*, meaning law or rule. Self-rule implies self-discipline and self-responsibility: The person who attributes his own (mis)conduct to others, who blames it on being a victim of circumstances, or who enlists the assistance of others in tasks he could perform for himself (such as self-care in general and suicide in particular) is diminishing his own autonomy. I shall return to this point later, when I consider the views of communitarian critics of autonomy.

Autonomy is not something we possess by virtue of biological nature (such as a pancreas) or by virtue of citizenship or personhood (such as the right to life, liberty, and the pursuit of happiness). As with liberty, autonomy is not something one person can give another, although one person can foster or frustrate another's autonomy. Because the behavioral-psychological basis of autonomy is the ability to control one's own conduct, it must be acquired and safeguarded by each person for himself. As with personal independence, autonomy is potentially increased by education, intelligence, and health and is often diminished by their absence. In the final analysis, however, autonomy rests on self-discipline. As Edmund Burke memorably phrased it: "Society cannot exist unless a controlling power upon will and appetite be placed somewhere, and the less there is within, the more there must be without. It is ordained in the eternal constitution of things, that men of intemperate minds cannot be free. Their passions forge their fetters."[9]

In ethics and philosophy, the term "autonomy" denotes, as *Webster's Dictionary* states, self-sufficiency. However, we are social creatures through and through. There is no such thing as an autonomous person; we are more or less autonomous, depending on circumstances and comparisons with others or with our own former or future selves. That does not render the term any less useful. However, it requires keeping in mind that our need for autonomy is intrinsically at odds with our need for relationship with other human beings (or with animals and imaginary or nonhuman beings endowed with human attributes). It also requires that we attribute autonomy only to *persons as individuals, never as members of a group*. It is a mistake to attribute autonomy to persons-in-relation, for example, as doctors or patients: It is as foolish to talk about "patient autonomy" as it would be to talk about "husband autonomy" or "wife autonomy." Each member of such a pair willingly enters into a *human bond*, the very point of which is to sacrifice some portion of his autonomy (independence), in exchange for some measure of security or service (dependence). Every relationship—to other persons, to deities, and even to pets—entails a measure of dependency and loss of autonomy. The very purpose of forming attachments is to love and be loved and to experience needing and being needed. Why else would men create God, if not to love Him and be loved by Him in return?

This goes a long way toward explaining why Judaism, Christianity, and Islam condemn suicide as the autonomous ending of one's own life. The conventional explanation—that the commandment "Thou shalt not kill" forbids it—is hedged by too many exceptions to do the job. It seems to me more plausible to interpret this prohibition as God's commanding man to never abandon Him, a directive explicitly stated in the Decalogue. Unlike the Greek gods who kept each other company, the Jewish God is alone in the world: He is married to Man and His greatest fear is divorce.

I am suggesting that man's invention of a God from whom he must never be separated and the prohibition of suicide arise from and satisfy the same basic need—the child's need never to be separated from his parent. The child's profound sense of dependence and need for protection leave a permanent trace in the human mind. The prohibition, "You must never leave me" and the promise it entails, "I shall never leave you"—communications often exchanged by lovers in precisely those terms—are the most effective reassurances we have against this basic anxiety. This interpretation is consistent with the suspension of the prohibition against suicide—indeed, its instant metamorphosis from sin into virtue—if the deed is perceived as an act of (timeless) *attachment* rather than (permanent) *detachment*: for example, being united with God (martyrdom) or with the beloved (double suicide à la Romeo and Juliet). Only when suicide is seen as the epitome of autonomy, as the ultimate *detachment* from God and other people, is it considered a sin and a crime (worse than murder).

Autonomy, Liberty, and Rights

Although the terms "autonomy" and "right" refer to radically different concepts, they are often confused and misused. *Autonomy* is self-directed (or, to use John Stuart Mill's phrase, "self-regarding"): It is exercising one's own powers to act in accordance with one's own free will, for example, resisting a temptation or yielding to it and assuming responsibility for the consequences. *Right* is other-directed ("other-regarding"): It is lodging a "rightful" claim against others or the State, for example, to payment for services rendered as contractually agreed upon.

This distinction is so important and is so often neglected, even by political philosophers, that it may be useful to restate it in somewhat different language. Political theorist Anthony de Jasay distinguishes between "liberties to perform" and "rights to performance." (De Jasay's "liberty to perform" is synonymous with the liberty to exercise one's autonomy.) He writes: "A right confers a benefit on its holder. In order for him to enjoy it, an obligor must fulfill the corollary obligation—which is generally onerous to a degree. . . . A liberty, on the other hand, is exercised without calling for specific performance by any other party; apart from negative externalities that may be generated by my using it, my liberty is costless to everybody else. . . . 'Costly to others' and 'costless to others' are no more alike than black and white."[10]

The situation with respect to the autonomy of the suicide is thus as follows: The voluntary death of a particular person may be cost-saving, costless, or costly (to family and society). When suicide is cost-saving or costless, there is no prudential reason for preventing or condemning it. When it is costly, it may be justifiable to condemn suicide and use persuasion to prevent it, but it is unjustifiable to resort to coercion to interfere with it. Actually, regardless of how disabled a person may be, as long as he is conscious he can kill himself, without (active) assistance, by refusing to eat. Everyone possesses this ultimate reservoir of autonomy, and virtually everyone recoils from acknowledging it.

The progress of civilization and the division of labor on which it rests foster as well as inhibit autonomy. Science and technology augment our powers of self-sustenance and self-care, but they also make us more dependent on physical artifacts and social networks of increasing complexity. Our lives are longer, healthier, and more secure than were the lives of our forebears, yet we seem more anxious about confronting the challenges of everyday life than they were. Never before have people been so overwrought about suicide as we are. Never before have people so insistently affirmed and denied, deified and demonized, the role free choice plays in voluntary death. One of the manifestations of this ambivalence and confusion is that American Medicine, Law, and popular opinion disapprove of suicide if it is carried out without *clinical imprimatur*, but approve of it if it is carried out with it. In the former case, it is viewed as a "treatable disease" to be forcibly prevented by doctors. In the latter case, it is viewed as a "compassionate treatment" to which certain medically identified individuals have a constitutional right.

Despite widespread opposition to and rejection of autonomous suicide and increasing acceptance of and support for medicalized "suicide," physicians, lawyers, and journalists maintain that autonomy is our supreme national value and that physicians promote and safeguard "patient autonomy." The following opinion by Timothy E. Quill and Howard Brody, two of the most respected writers on medical ethics, is typical. Quill and Brody are not satisfied with respecting persons as moral agents, endowed with rights and responsibilities. They believe that persons as patients need something more and to that end they propose an "enhanced autonomy model [which] allows the physician to support and guide the patient without surrendering the medical power on which the patient depends."[11] What they mean by "enhanced autonomy" is this: "Other moral considerations may override an individual patient's *right to autonomous choice or even to participate in the decision. Justice may demand that one patient is not given what is individually optimal because another patient has a greater moral entitlement to a scarce resource.* . . . Mental competence must be assured before patients can be allowed to make decisions that appear to be against their own best interests (for example, a suicidal patient who wants to be discharged probably should not be)."[12] In other words, a patient has "enhanced autonomy" when physicians deprive him of his *"right to autonomous choice"* to satisfy the needs of *"another patient [who] has a greater moral entitlement to a scarce resource."* This statement requires no further comment.

Being terminally ill in a hospital, much less being on a ventilator, reduces the subject's autonomy to the vanishing point. That may be one of the reasons why writers of end-of-life decisions vociferously proclaim their devotion to "patient autonomy," believe that some patients have a "right to physician-assisted suicide," and insist that, despite the fact that the term "physician-assisted suicide" contains the word, *physician-assisted suicide is not suicide.* Helping such a person die—indirectly, by disconnecting life-sustaining treatment, or directly, by "euthanizing" him—may or may not be morally blameworthy or praiseworthy. But that is not the point. The point is that such acts have nothing to do with the patient's autonomy. Nor are those acts suicide (or physician-assisted suicide), even if they are carried out at the request of and with the consent of the patient. A physician who removes a patient from life support with the patient's consent performs a deed that may, morally, be comparable to placing the patient on life support with the patient's consent. In each case, the patient is the principal and the physician is his agent. If the patient authorizes the physician to remove his life support, then the act is an instance of *justifiable medical homi-*

cide; if the patient does not authorize it, then it is an instance of *unjustifiable medical homicide*.

Medical killing is medical killing. It exists and we ought to have an adequate vocabulary for describing its various forms. Medical killing has nothing to do with autonomy. A ventilator supporting a person's respiration is like a beam supporting a platform: Remove the support and the object it supports—the human body or the platform—collapses. If a patient discontinues his own life support—as do some patients on hemodialysis, about which I shall say more presently—then he terminates his own life: He kills himself (autohomicide). Conversely, if someone else discontinues a patient's life support—which is the case with patients on mechanical ventilators—then that person terminates the patient's life: He kills another person (heterohomicide).

The physician who takes a patient off a ventilator is undoing the earlier act of placing him on it. If we view maintaining a patient on life support as "giving" him life, then we should have the courage to view removing him from life support as "taking his life" (a life the patient would continue to have, at least for a while longer, were he to remain on life support). If we cannot accept such "mercy killing," we ought to abstain from using medical technology, which would be foolish, since some persons placed on life support recover to live without it. We struggle with these dilemmas not only because they are morally weighty, but also because we lack a vocabulary for some of the ways people die nowadays—and also because we lack the courage to speak clearly and assume responsibility for our actions.

The Communitarian War on Autonomy

When I was a young physician, before the phony egalitarianism of medical correctness deformed and dominated medical discourse, doctors acknowledged their domination over patients as sick persons in need of authoritative guidance; their arrogance was tempered by candor. Today, physicians disguise their domination over patients by attributing autonomy to them; their arrogance masquerades as concern for "patient rights." The result is that the contemporary medical literature on the doctor-patient relationship is largely cant. By calling benevolent paternalism "patient autonomy," the "experts" systematically obscure the fundamental antagonism between authority and autonomy and misrepresent subordination-submission as cooperation.

A Latin legal maxim reminds us of an important truth: "*Nullum crimen majus est inobedientia*" (No crime is greater than disobedience).[13] Some years ago, I rephrased this adage as follows: "There is only one offense against authority: self-control; and only one obeisance to it: submission to control by authority."[14] It is folly to pretend that these principles do not apply to the relationship between the physician as a superior and the patient as a subordinate.

The person who controls himself and cares for his own well-being has no need of, or tolerance for, an authority as *his protector from himself*. He is his own self-protector, which renders paternalistic authority unemployed. What is he to do if he cannot control others in the name of protecting them? He could mind his own business. But that is a fatuous answer. Persons satisfied with minding their own business do not aspire to become paternalistic authorities, while persons who become such authorities consider minding other people's business their own business and call it "caring" and "assuming responsibility." Authority thus needs persons who lack autonomy or whom they can readily deprive of it (children, old people, and patients). Hence, the ceaseless warfare of authority against autonomy, "against suicide, against masturbation, against self-medication, against the proper use of language itself."[15]

Perhaps nothing is more revealing of the contemporary American medical attitude toward autonomy than that both friends and foes of physician-assisted suicide (PAS) oppose autonomous physician-unassisted suicide (PUS) and support coercive psychiatric suicide prevention (CPSP). The friends of PAS object to PUS because they believe that only a person vetted by psychiatrists and declared "not depressed" ought to have a right to take his own life. The foes of PAS oppose suicide *per se* and hence PAS as well, because they believe that these acts injure the community and therefore no one has a right to die voluntarily. Self-declared communitarian Wesley J. Smith writes: "[C]ommunitarianism promotes mutual interpersonal care, concern, and support. Communitarianism *mandates that the state prevent harm to the weak and vulnerable—for example, by stopping suicides*—not as a loathsome act of paternalism but as an act of human obligation to protect and care for one another."[16] Note that Smith is not satisfied with advancing "care, concern, and support" as justifications for using state-sanctioned coercions to protect people from themselves; he also claims that such benevolent coercion is *not* an "act of paternalism."

It is revealing that Smith rests his opposition to suicide on the Zulu concept *ubutu*, a notion, he explains, that "has no exact English counterpart . . . but can roughly be translated as being all the attributes that go into that exquisite spark that makes *humankind* special and unique in the known universe. . . . When we stand by and watch . . . profiteers threatening the well-being of patients, we are losing our *ubutu*. . . . Will we choose to love each other or abandon each other? The bottom line is: Will we keep or lose our *ubutu*?"[17] The danger of losing our *ubutu* is admittedly a novel justification for psychiatric coercion in the name of suicide prevention.

By training and by practice, physicians tend to be paternalists, and psychiatrists tend to be coercive paternalists: They are prone to misconstrue autonomy as hostility to the community, especially the community of patients. Shimon M. Glick, M.D., a physician at Ben Gurion University in Israel, credits Judaism for inculcating these values into physicians and views CPSP, perfected by non-Jewish psychiatrists in the nineteenth century, as the expression of a specifically Jewish virtue.[18] He writes:

Israeli medical ethics deviates considerably from Western norms. . . . The biblical admonition "Do not stand idly by your friend's blood" creates an imperative for extensive involvement in the affairs of others, for their benefit. . . . In addition, the concept of mutual responsibility among Jews has been clearly articulated: "All Jews are responsible for each other's deeds."* . . . The traditional Jewish view says, "You are so valuable to us, beyond what you mean to yourself, that we simply cannot permit you to die. We care so much about you that *we are willing even to violate your human rights in order to save your life.*"

Glick proudly reports having administered court-ordered "force-feeding [to] a group of political prisoners engaged in a hunger strike" and cites the case of an orthodox Jew who "requested assurance that the tube feedings meet his particular high standards of kosher food and that he be permitted to deposit a letter, with copies sent to a list of government authorities, indicating that he was being fed against his express wishes and that I [Glick] would bear the legal and criminal consequences. When this was accomplished, he offered no resistance." Glick reassures us that he does not "countenance the complicity of physicians with totalitarian regimes when they force-feed fasting protesters." He does not say whether, for example, the British authorities acted laudably or lamentably when they refrained from force-feeding Gandhi.

Daniel Callahan, a prominent medical ethicist, believes that Americans have too much autonomy and opposes physician-assisted suicide because it augments individual self-determination. I, too, oppose it, not because it expands personal autonomy, but because it diminishes it (and for other reasons as well). Callahan states: "What we are trying to do with assisted suicide is to take a step beyond which there are no other steps in *gaining full individual self-determination*. . . . If autonomy is the greatest moral good, we will have an impoverished, self-involved society. . . . Asking for this *ultimate control* does great harm to the individual and to society."[19] Callahan confuses other-determination (intrinsic to PAS, with the physician as superior

---

*This passage resembles the Deuteronomic injunction requiring Jews to treat Jews and non-Jews differently. Glick classifies his views as "communitarian" and adds: "It is perhaps no coincidence that one of the chief proponents of the communitarian movement in the United States is a former Israeli [Amitai Etzioni]."

and the patient as his subordinate) with self-determination (exercised by persons who commit suicide without physician assistance).[20] Legalizing PAS gives more control to physicians, not to patients. Because autonomy implies assuming responsibility for satisfying one's needs and taking responsibility for one's actions, its expansion leads to a less self-involved and more harmonious society. Legalizing PAS is not a step toward more self-determination for patients; it is a step toward intensified medical-statist tutelage for everyone as potential patient.

A similar revolt against (excessive) individualism animates the antisuicide zeal of Willard Gaylin and Bruce Jennings, the authors of *The Perversion of Autonomy*, candidly subtitled: *The Proper Uses of Coercion and Constraints in a Liberal Society*. Gaylin is a psychiatrist and a prominent medical ethicist. Jennings is the executive director of the Hastings Center, a think tank devoted to exploring contemporary issues of medical ethics. Although I disagree with Gaylin and Jennings's views on autonomy, I share many of their concerns about the dangers that obsession with the self, epitomized by the cult of self-esteem, poses to the integrity of society. Whereas Gaylin and Jennings oppose PAS because it caters excessively to autonomy, I oppose it, among other reasons, because it undermines and diminishes autonomy.

The concepts of mental illness and personal autonomy are antithetical: The more people believe in the reality of the former, the more they distrust the value of the latter, and vice versa. Gaylin and Jennings's thesis rests heavily on the traditional psychiatric denial of free will, choice, and rational suicide. They state: "Human behavior is less rational than most of us would like to believe. . . . [It] is less 'voluntary' than libertarians and theorists of autonomy would have it. Present behavior is significantly determined by past treatment."[21] These are truisms with no bearing on the nature or value of autonomy. They do, however, effectively obscure the important conceptual, legal, and political differences between verbal persuasion and physical coercion.

Instead of refuting autonomy as a useful philosophical concept and estimable moral value, Gaylin and Jennings assault it, asserting that autonomy "now preempts civility, altruism, paternalism, beneficence, community, mutual aid, and other moral values that essentially tell the person to set aside his own interests in favor of the interests of other people or the good of something larger than himself."[22] This is a gross distortion of the meaning of autonomy, which the authors themselves *correctly identify as "the state of being self-governed or self-sovereign."*[23] Being self-governed encourages rather than discourages civility: The autonomous person governed by reason is more likely to be open-minded and generous toward his fellow man than is the heteronomous person governed by envy and xenophobia.[24]

The basic reason Gaylin and Jennings cavil about Americans' having too much autonomy is because they equate autonomy with childish willfulness, and because, like the supporters of PAS whose views they reject, they believe that "the right to active assistance with committing suicide" enhances autonomy. They write: "[T]aking the logic of autonomy one step further, does it mean the patient has a *right to active assistance with committing suicide? Must physician-assisted suicide and euthanasia be legalized . . . or can autonomy be overridden here in the name of competing social values and interests?* These social values include respecting the sanctity of life, protecting those who are vulnerable to medical abuse and neglect."[25]

It is not clear what Gaylin and Jennings mean by "sanctity of life." It is an emotionally charged phrase whose meaning is obscured by its regular use as a religious-political slogan. Although they approvingly cite St. Paul, for whom "perfect freedom was perfect servitude, albeit in the service of Christ,"[26] they do not claim to be writing as Christian ethicists, some of whom condemn autonomy as a rejection of dependence on God and "withdrawal from humanity into a private, meaningless world."[27] If Gaylin and Jennings's views rest on such a religious premise, they ought to say so, in which case they must condemn suicide *ab ovo* and need no further argument against PAS. However, if they write as secular medical ethicists, then their respect for the sanctity of life must include respect for the sanctity of death as well. Dying, after all, belongs to the living, not to the dead.

Disregarding the deprivations of autonomy entailed by the war on drugs, the countless uses of psychiatric excuses and coercions in everyday life, and the numerous regulations imposed on Americans by the myriad alphabet agencies of the government, Gaylin and Jennings declare: "Creating a society in which autonomy flourishes has been one of America's greatest achievements."[28] Alas, if that were only true.

STOPPING LIFE BY STOPPING LIFE SUPPORT

One of the consequences of advances in medical technology is that increasing numbers of persons can be kept alive, for short or long periods, by machines that perform some of their vital functions. The use of such machines—for example, for hemodialysis and mechanical ventilation—has created the possibility of ending one's own life or a patient's life by disconnecting the machine. That option has led not only to debates about the dilemmas thus created, but also to attempts to justify physician-assisted suicide (PAS) and voluntary euthanasia (VE) by analogizing them with taking patients off life support. Along the way, everyone seems to have lost sight of the fact that—morally, legally, and logically—the problem of suicide is anterior to the problems of discontinuing life support, PAS, and VE. As long as we are unsure about where we stand on *suicide per se* (that is, *physician-unassisted suicide*)—as long as we are undecided about whether it is *a moral choice or a medical problem*, whether it is or ought to be *legal or illegal*—we cannot rationally analyze the arguments for and against PAS and VE.

The patient on dialysis is physically able to discontinue being dialyzed. If he does so, is he committing suicide? If this appears to be a difficult question, it is not because the concept of voluntary death (autohomicide) is ambiguous, but because our discourse about it is linguistically so impoverished and distorted that we are unable to speak about *nonstigmatizing voluntary death*. Instead, we intensify mutilating the English language by insisting that deliberate, voluntary self-destruction is "not suicide." In the official "Opinion" of the American Medical Association, "withdrawal of life-sustaining treatment which allows the patient to die of the primary disease is neither suicide nor assisted suicide."[29] However, such a death is phenomenologically different from the death of a patient who continues life-sustaining treatment and dies of a complication of the treatment or, finally, of the primary disease itself. Moreover, such a death, induced voluntarily by the individual who wants to end his life, is clearly an act of autohomicide. The fact that we have deliberately avoided distinguishing between justifiable and unjustifiable suicide and have thus deprived ourselves from classifying some deaths as cases of "justifiable suicide" proves only that we have crippled our language, not that stopping dialysis is "not suicide."

Suicide by Discontinuing Hemodialysis

The artificial kidney was developed in 1944, primarily for the treatment of *acute* renal shutdown. In the 1960s, hemodialysis began to be used as a treatment for *chronic* end-stage kidney disease. Since 1973, government insurance programs have covered the cost of this form of maintenance therapy. Today, hundreds of thousands of persons the world over depend on hemodialysis for their survival, which is both a blessing and a curse.

The patient on dialysis must spend about 20 hours per week attached to the machinery that rids his body of metabolites, must adhere to a strict diet, and is certain to experience many debilitating physical symptoms and social problems. The longer he stays on dialysis, the more the quality of his life deteriorates. Chad H. Calland, a physician-victim of end-stage renal disease, thought it doubtful that many patients would begin hemodialysis if they knew how poor the quality of their lives would be once they are on it. He lamented also that should a patient come to this conclusion, he would run the risk of being declared and treated as mentally ill. He wrote: "Many of these conflicts are considered by most psychiatrists to be evidence of depressive or paranoid ideation. I cannot emphasize strongly enough that, in this group of patients, these fears are well founded and are based on reality. ... Is it necessary to postulate psychiatric disorders to understand the self-evident?"[30] Calland evidently failed to realize that, in our culture, the only thing about suicide that is self-evident is that it is *due to treatable depression.*

Joseph T. DiBianco, a professor of psychiatry at New York Medical College who has worked with hemodialysis patients, writes: "The daily stresses under which hemodialysis patients live should be sufficient to forewarn us that some patients will be unable and/or unwilling to cope with this regimen. Thus suicidal behaviors can be expected to occur with a high frequency among the dialysis population."[31] So-called suicidal behavior is estimated to be 100 to 400 times more frequent in patients on hemodialysis than in the general population.[32] Most psychiatrists regard noncompliance with dialysis as a symptom of depression and suicidality; most nephrologists do not.[33] Because there is basic disagreement about what counts as suicide in dialysis patients, the statistics about voluntary death among such patients is unreliable. Statistics about voluntarily discontinuing dialysis are another matter.

Studies show that whites, the elderly, and diabetics withdraw from dialysis more often than do blacks, the young, and nondiabetics. In English-speaking countries, voluntary withdrawal from dialysis is the second most frequent cause of death among such patients (second only to heart disease). In Australia about 30 percent and in the United States about 20 percent of the deaths in dialysis patients are due to withdrawal.[34] In non-English-speaking countries, death caused by withdrawal from dialysis is much less common or is less commonly reported or so classified.[35] Two Italian nephrologists state: "Our clinical impression is that death from suicide and treatment termination is a rare event among Renal Replacement Therapy [hemodialysis] patients in Italy."[36] The reasons may lie in less frequent recourse to dialysis, differences in patient selection and reporting practices, and cultural dissimilarities.

There is an instructive similarity between the patient who kills himself by discontinuing hemodialysis and the person who kills himself by ingesting a lethal drug. Both possess the chemicals needed for committing suicide: In the first case, the subject's own body manufactures the chemicals; in the second case, a pharmaceutical company does. The difference between suicide by discontinuing dialysis and suicide by conventional means is essentially a difference of means. Although suicide by discontinuing hemodialysis may appear to be an act of omission and suicide by ingesting a drug an act of commission, both types of voluntary death are actually acts of commission. We may choose to judge the two acts as morally different, but phenomenologically both are instances of deliberate, voluntary death (autohomicide). Some people may object that only some persons have the opportunity to kill themselves by discontinuing dialysis. True, but only some persons have the opportunity to kill themselves by ingesting barbiturates or shooting themselves. The defining element in suicide is not the method used, but the *deliberate action* to bring it about. To be sure, just as not every killing of others is deliberate, not every self-killing is deliberate. Accordingly, we must distinguish between deliberate and accidental suicide, not declare that voluntarily discontinuing dialysis or some other life-sustaining procedure is "not suicide."

Deliberate action is the basic feature that is shared not only by contraception and suicide, but also by the countless deliberate actions—good, bad, and indifferent—in which we engage. We call the decision to create or not create life "birth control" and ought to call the decision to leave or not leave life "death control."[37] As long as we reject that (or some similar) semantic option, we shall be unable to abandon our traditional prejudices against suicide.

Notwithstanding the similarities between suicide by discontinuing dialysis and suicide by more direct means, the reactions of nephrologists and psychiatrists to these acts, respectively, could hardly be more different. Nephrologists accept that a person may consider dying preferable to living tethered to a dialysis machine and they believe they "should honor a competent patient's request or an incompetent patient's clearly expressed prior wishes [to discontinue dialysis]."[38] Psychiatrists who work on dialysis units also accept this type of suicide; nevertheless they are eager to preserve the privilege of deciding who will be allowed to discontinue dialysis and who will not. Lewis M. Cohen, a Massachusetts psychiatrist, writes: "When I determine that a dialysis cessation request is motivated by depression or other forms of psychopathology, I have not hesitated to institute vigorous psychiatric treatment, including hospital commitment."[39] In contrast and despite Bleuler's classic warning,[40] psychiatrists are unwilling to accept that living tethered to the institution of psychiatry may be just as intolerable as living tethered to a dialysis machine. They believe that a suicidal person's wish to die directly—rather than by refusing a life-sustaining treatment—should *never* be honored; moreover, they have persuaded the law that they, the psychiatrists, ought to be obligated to prevent such a person's suicide, by force if necessary.

There is another difference between the nephrologists' relationship with patients maintained on dialysis and the psychiatrists' relationship with patients maintained on antipsychotic drug treatment. Occasionally, nephrologists must deal with patients who want to continue dialysis even though their physicians consider further treatment "futile" and "irrational." To put it bluntly, nephrologists sometimes encounter patients who, they believe, ought to die by withdrawing from dialysis but who refuse to do so. In a report titled, "Competent patients, incompetent decisions," three Australian nephrologists describe the case of a 70-year-old woman "with end-stage renal failure and terminal malignancy who wanted to continue dialysis even though those caring for her considered this choice irrational. . . . [To the staff,] respecting her wishes by continuing dialysis appeared to be both expensive and futile." After wrestling with the issue of "patient autonomy," the authors concluded that "there are arguments for overriding patients' wishes when they conflict with medical opinion." The physicians discontinued dialyzing the patient. "Autonomy," they explained, "may also be restricted if the physician believes that a patient would be harmed by the requested treatment."[41]

These writers assume that persons called "physicians" have, and ought to have, the *legal right* to restrict the autonomy of their patients. As noted earlier in this chapter, that is not the case if the patient is more powerful than the physician; if, by virtue of his economic or political power, the patient is the superior and the doctor is his subordinate. The more physicians take their superior position toward their patients for granted, the more they lose sight of how their tacit assumptions about their own and their patients' economic and existential situations affect their ethical judgments and clinical decisions.

For obvious reasons, psychiatrists do not face this problem: They never encounter "psychotic" (depressed or schizophrenic) patients who, in the opinion of their physicians, are so hopelessly sick and untreatable that they ought to discontinue the use of antipsychotic drugs (and kill themselves), but who refuse to stop taking the drugs (that ostensibly prevent them from killing themselves).

Finally, nephrologists occasionally encounter dialysis patients whose treatment they (the doctors) want to stop because the patients persistently sabotage treatment (by nonadherence to diet, drug abuse, and so forth) and whose disruptive behavior interferes with the operation of the dialysis unit. Because declaring such persons mentally ill and dangerous to themselves would merely add a psychiatric diagnosis to the patient's record but would not solve the doctors' dilemma, nephrologists tend to cope with this problem by petitioning the court to permit them to discontinue dialysis. The typical result is a complex legal process, the patient usually dying before the controversy reaches a legal resolution.[42] Psychiatrists never face this sort of dilemma: They never encounter depressed or schizophrenic patients whose treatment with antipsychotic drugs they (the doctors) want to stop because the patients persistently sabotage the treatment (by noncompliance with taking the medication, drug abuse, and so forth) and whose disruptive behavior interferes with the operation of the psychiatric unit. The point, of course, is not that psychiatrists do not have to deal with such patients, but that they deal with them by intensifying the coercions that pass as "treatments" in psychiatry.

It must be emphasized that nephrologists enjoy powerful support for their tolerant posture toward letting patients as well as physicians discontinue dialysis: The American Medical Association (AMA) and the bioethics community endorse the fiction that killing oneself by stopping dialysis is *not suicide*, that this mode of dying is identical to dying from the primary disease. As mentioned earlier, the official AMA "Opinion" on life-sustaining therapy concludes with this comforting assertion: "Withdrawal of life-sustaining treatment [such as dialysis] is neither suicide nor assisted suicide." This assertion flies in the face of common sense, of the dictionary definition of suicide, and of the psychiatric classification of self-starvation in anorexia nervosa as a type of suicide.

Surely it is fair to compare deliberate withdrawal from the life-sustaining procedure of dialysis in renal disease with deliberate withdrawal from the life-sustaining procedure of eating in anorexia nervosa. Is such refusal of food a form of suicide? The authoritative *Comprehensive Textbook of Psychiatry—II*, states: "Some psychiatrists have considered anorexia nervosa as a variant of suicide."[43] Hilde Bruch, an internationally recognized expert on anorexia nervosa, wrote: "Anorexia nervosa has been referred to as 'suicide in refracted doses.' "[44]

The difference between a physically ill person discontinuing dialysis and a physically healthy person discontinuing eating is not that one *is not* suicide and the other *is*, but that we approve of the former and disapprove of the latter. It would be better simply to say so and stop playing games with the language of how we die.

Further Reflections on the Semantics of Suicide

I realize that bioethicists object to the view that discontinuing dialysis—and, generally, discontinuing life-sustaining treatment (LST) of any kind—is a type of suicide: They maintain that such a patient dies of his primary disease. However, if the patient were to continue LST, he would not die (when he dies). How badly or how much longer he would live are important considerations for justifying the decision to stop LST; but they do not negate the fact that the proximal cause of death is suicide (autohomicide). To demonstrate that this conclusion is logically inevitable, all we need to do is change the scenario a little.

Suppose that a dialysis patient discontinues his treatment and a few days later is killed by an intruder: His death would be considered murder (heterohomicide), and the person who caused it would be classified as a murderer. The fact that the length of life forfeited by the suicide of the sick person on LST is shorter than that forfeited by the suicide of the healthy person is beside the point. The point is that, in each case, the subject's deliberate action is the proximal cause of his own death. Both the person who causes himself to die by discontinuing LST and the person who causes himself to die by ingesting an overdose of a sedative *dies when and as he wants to die* instead of waiting to die in a manner and at a time not of his own choosing. Phenomenologically, both types of death are instances of autohomicide. Morally, we may want to—and perhaps ought to—distinguish one from another. However, we do not claim that because a homicide is justifiable (say, because it is self-defense), it is "not homicide." By the same token, we ought not claim that because a suicide is justifiable (say, because it is self-defense against a physically invasive and existentially injurious medical treatment), it is "not suicide." It would be better to enrich our vocabulary so that we could identify some cases of suicide *as* suicide, without stigmatizing the actor, and validate the act without denying its true nature.

Once a person undertakes a life-sustaining treatment, it requires an act of commission on his part to stop it. In other words, the essential difference between the suicide of a person who kills himself indirectly by discontinuing LST and the suicide of a person who kills himself directly is not simply the difference between omission and commission. The difference is that we accept the former as morally valid and reject the latter as morally invalid. This point is dramatically illustrated by the comments provoked by the death of the renowned writer James Michener. On October 3, 1997, the newspapers reported that Michener, aged 90, "has taken himself off life-sustaining kidney dialysis. . . . An unnamed source [stated] 'He's decided he doesn't want to go on living like this.' "[45]

"Did James Michener commit suicide or just die?" asked Bruce Hilton, director of the National Center for Bioethics. "After all those years of advocating a moral core for life, did he end up thumbing his nose at morality and the law?" No, said Hilton. What Michener did "is called allowing to die or letting nature take its course. It is 'withdrawing inappropriate treatment,' 'right to refuse treatment,' or 'passive euthanasia.' *One thing it's not is suicide.*"[46]

Hilton wants to think well of Michener, which Michener richly deserves; hence he cannot bring himself to say that Michener committed suicide. In other words, Hilton rejects attributing a descriptive-phenomenological, nonstigmatizing meaning to the term "suicide": He cannot give up believing that committing suicide is synonymous with moral failure or mental illness or both. Given that constraint, Hilton is compelled to call Michener's voluntary death *"not suicide."*

Ironically, in his effort to excuse Michener from an act that needs no excuse, Hilton demeans Michener by denying that he died as a responsible moral agent and that his death was admirable. Instead, Hilton perceives and presents Michener as a helpless victim of circumstances. He writes: "He [Michener] was in an artificial situation, kept from *natural death* by the intricacies of medical technology." Michener was not "kept" from natural death. When he went on dialysis, he *decided* to keep himself from dying from the "natural" cause of kidney failure (prevented by "artificial" dialysis); when he went off dialysis, he *decided* to die of kidney failure, a "natural death" (instead of, say, a stroke, which is also "natural" and is a common cause of death in patients on dialysis).

Finally, if Hilton considers dying from renal failure *natural* and therefore virtuous, than he must consider living on hemodialysis *unnatural* and therefore wicked. If this is how confused the director of the National Center for Bioethics is about what is and what is not "natural" or a "suicide," it is small wonder that the press and the public are confused about suicide. Hilton's saying that Michener did not commit suicide because his act was justified is like saying that Adolf Eichmann's executioners did not commit homicide because their deed was justified. *Webster's Dictionary* defines suicide as "an act or an instance of taking one's own life voluntarily and intentionally," and homicide as "the killing of one human being by another."

BIRTH AND DEATH: THE DIVINE/SATANIC SYMMETRY

Read as a cautionary tale, the gist of Genesis is the familiar admonition, "Don't get too big for your britches!" Life is God's business, not man's. The writers of the Bible dramatize man's quest for knowledge as a battle between God and Satan. God is the rightful governor of life and death. Man's aspiration to gain control over himself, over his own life and death, is tantamount to wresting control from God. Autonomy is *lèse majesté*. We call God the "Creator," Satan, the "Destroyer." Birth is Divine. Death is Satanic.*

Controlling Birth and Death: Prohibition, Medicalization, and the Repeal of Prohibition

Unimpeded by human intelligence and interference, reproduction (in man and many animals) is the *unintended* consequence of copulation, while death is the *unintended* consequence of being eaten by another animal or succumbing to disease, injury, or old age. For eons, the lives and deaths of human beings were governed by these seemingly inviolable laws of biology. However, at some point in the dim past, people recognized the connec-

---

*These are Jewish and Christian images. The Hindu-Buddhist concept of nirvana celebrates death as a permanent state of being as not-being. For Hindus and Buddhists, suicide is a fearful option because it guarantees painful reincarnation.

tion between coitus and conception. This momentous discovery gave them a measure of control over procreation: by abstinence, masturbation, homosexuality, contraception, and abortion. Causing death by killing must have been a much earlier discovery.

In short, we have long ago wrested from God the right to kill others as well as the right to control our own powers of reproduction. But we continue to fear wresting from Him the power to control our own death. To be sure, we are creeping up on Him. We say it is permissible to "hasten" a "natural death," that is, a death He has already prepared for us. But it is not permissible to choose the time and manner of our dying, regardless of His or of other authorities' approval or disapproval. It is an odd timidity. We go about our daily rounds as if it were none of His business where and how we live, yet we are afraid to declare that it is also none of His business when and how we die. Even worse, we deify doctors and delegate the power to regulate death to them.

God had good reasons to prohibit contraception and suicide. He created man to keep Him company, not to be deserted by him.[47] The life of early man was precarious and short. His collective mind, so to speak, recognized that contraception and suicide pose grave dangers to the survival of the group. Accordingly, he created gods to prohibit individuals from engaging in such "unnatural" acts. Fertility rites and taboos against suicide are consistent features of primitive religions; the injunctions to "multiply" and "not kill" are basic to the great Western monotheistic religions.

Ancient prohibitions against controlling birth and death imply that people correctly recognized that exercising that ability poses a threat to the group: Until relatively recently, most children died during infancy and most adults lived barely long enough to reproduce. Only since science has contributed to making life healthier and longer has birth control become a solution for the problem of poverty and overpopulation. Today, the prohibitions against birth control and death control no longer serve any prudential, sociobiological purpose. Moreover, although tradition and religion no longer control contraception, they still control suicide, although by medicalization rather than by theologization or criminalization.

Regrettably, our memory of the history of medicalization is short and selective: We remember its glories and forget its infamies, especially as they relate to sexual behavior. When I was born, contraception was under complete medical control and abortion was illegal. When I was an intern in a Boston hospital, offering contraceptive advice, much less providing a contraceptive device, was a criminal offense. Only in 1965, in the celebrated case of *Griswold v. Connecticut*, did the Supreme Court strike down as unconstitutional the statute that made it a crime for a person to "artificially prevent conception."[48] In that landmark case, the Court repealed the law that prohibited a conduct the law deemed illegal. It did not medicalize the alleged "condition" that motivates such conduct: The Court did not call the fear of pregnancy and the desire to avoid it a "disease," nor did it call engaging in the formerly prohibited conduct "physician-assisted contraception" or classify it as a "treatment." In short, the right to practice contraception was placed in the hands of the people, not in the hands of physicians.

Abortion underwent a similar metamorphosis, from sin to crime to right, with a brief stop-over as a treatment. When abortion was legalized, the mental illness whose treatment justified therapeutic abortion vanished. When suicide is legalized, the mental illness whose treatment justifies its therapeutic prevention will also vanish.

Although performing an abortion and developing effective methods of birth control entail the use of medical knowledge and skill, abortion and contraception are *not medical matters*. The same is true for suicide. Although killing oneself with a drug entails the use of medical knowledge and requires access to the necessary substance, *suicide is not a medical matter*. We ought to deal with death control the same way we have dealt with birth control: by removing it from the purview of Medicine and the State, by repealing all medical and legal interference with the act.

THE RIGHT TO DEATH CONTROL

Contemporary critics of the medical and moral legitimacy of suicide make two similar arguments: They define suicide as an illness and thus deny that it is an act; or they acknowledge that it is an act but deny that it is "rational" or "truly voluntary," annulling the moral significance of their acknowledgment. These attitudes are emblematic of suicide being our single most important social taboo: If a person wants to be accepted by society as "normal," he *must* question the mental competence of the suicide. We cannot rethink suicide without transcending this taboo.

From Vice to Virtue: Masturbation, Homosexuality, Suicide

The view that masturbators and homosexuals are not depraved or diseased is a recent development. Not long ago, psychiatric theory informed and justified the therapeutic persecution of persons who engaged in such behaviors, especially if psychiatrists attached the appropriate "diagnoses" to them.

The view that practicing birth control is a virtue rather than a vice is also a recent development. It took a long time for the opinion-makers of society to acknowledge that excessive procreation not only burdens parents, but also injures the very children whose welfare parents and society seek to promote. Only in this century did the practice of birth control become a hallmark of advanced societies. Even people who believe in religions that only yesterday forbade birth control now practice contraception and regard it as an act of responsible planning for the future.

We have rid ourselves of these false beliefs and the pernicious practices based on them, and we have effectively barred the State and its psychiatric agents from interfering with persons who engage in such behaviors. I submit that it is time to rid ourselves of the false belief that voluntary death is a moral wrong or the manifestation of a mental disorder. It is time to prohibit the State and its psychiatric agents from interfering with persons who engage in such behaviors. I feel confident that some day people will look back at our present prohibitory policies toward suicide with the same amazed disapproval with which we look back at our past prohibitory policies toward masturbation, homosexuality, and birth control.

Because we collectively approve of birth control, we do not automatically impugn a person's competence to practice contraception, and we do not try to interfere with his behavior on the ground that he is not competent to decide about so vital a matter. Conversely, because we collectively disapprove of suicide, we automatically impugn a person's competence to practice death control and interfere coercively with his behavior on precisely that ground. Although the deleterious consequences for society of impulsive, irresponsible procreation are far greater than are the deleterious consequences of impulsive, irresponsible suicide, we treat the opportunity to procreate, but not the opportunity to practice death control, as if it were an inalienable right. If we regard the coercive regulation of birth control as morally odious and legally impermissible, as indeed we should, then we ought to regard the coercive regulation of death control as even more odious and impermissible.

Death Control: The Last Option and Final Responsibility

What did the writers of the Bible mean when they wrote: "To every thing there is a season, and a time to every purpose under the heaven: A time to be born, and a time to die"?

I believe they meant to remind us that life is a relentless cycle of birth, growth, decline, and death. As there comes a time when a woman is too old to have a child, so there comes a time when we may be too disabled to kill ourselves. The woman who does not want to end up childless must have a baby while she can, perhaps earlier than she might feel ready to do so. Similarly, if we do not want to die a lingering death after a protracted period of pathetic disability, we must kill ourselves while we can, perhaps earlier than we might feel ready to do so.

We are not responsible for being born. But from the moment we acquire the power of self-reflection, we are, increasingly as we age, responsible for how we live—and how we die. The option of killing oneself is intrinsic to human life (except during early childhood and sometimes in old age). We are born involuntarily. Religion, psychiatry, and the State insist that we die the same way. *That is what makes dying voluntarily the ultimate freedom.* We have just as much right and responsibility to regulate how we die as we have to regulate how we live. To be sure, suicidal activity, like any intimate bodily activity, ought to be permissible only in private. Public suicidal activity, exemplified by a person's threatening to jump from a high building, interferes with the everyday activities of others, constitutes a public nuisance, and ought to be prohibited and punished by the criminal law.

Rights and responsibilities, as I have emphasized, are not behaviors that persons have independently of other persons; they are attributes that characterize and belong to persons in relation to other persons. It takes two responders to generate responsibilities.* We should not hold a person responsible, nor should he hold himself responsible, for bringing about an event he cannot control, for example, the sunset. Similarly, we should not hold a person responsible, nor should he hold himself responsible, for not performing an act that the law prohibits, for example, killing himself with an illegal drug. However, we should hold a person responsible, and he should hold himself responsible, for doing things that he can control. Prohibiting death control—like prohibiting birth control, drug use, and other self-regarding behaviors—reduces the individual's opportunities to assume responsibility for the prohibited behaviors and makes the person dependent on external controls instead of on self-control. Therein lies the most insidious danger of relying on external prohibitions to regulate behaviors that can, in the final analysis, be effectively regulated *only* by internal controls. If young people believe that they cannot, need not, or must not control how they procreate—because assuming such control is wrong (sinful) and/or because others will assume responsibility for the consequences of their nonaction—then they are likely to create new life irresponsibly. Similarly, if old people believe that they cannot, need not, or must not control how they die—because assuming such control is wrong (a mental illness) and/or because others will assume responsibility for the consequences of their nonaction—then they are likely to die irresponsibly.

I do not mean that we have a responsibility to commit suicide (for example, when we are a burden to ourselves and those around us) or that we have a right to suicide (except in the weak sense of the word "right," meaning that agents of the State ought to be prohibited from forcibly preventing

---

*This is not literally true. We can hold ourselves responsible. The term then refers to an imaginary split between the individual as actor and as judge of his own action.

suicide). I am neither praising and recommending nor condemning and discouraging suicide, in the abstract. What I am saying is, simply, that:

- We have a choice and hence a responsibility between staying the course, living until death claims us, or quitting before it does, by killing ourselves.

- This choice and responsibility is similar to the choice and responsibility for staying single and getting married, or staying childless and having children.

- We ought to debate and resolve the problem of physician-prevented suicide *before* we engage in debating or legislating about physician-provided suicide.

Supporters and opponents of the "right to treatment," the "right to die," the "right to physician-assisted suicide," and similarly sloganized "rights" do not limit themselves to arguing their cause. They also litigate in the courts and lobby politicians to impose, with the power of the Therapeutic State unconstrained by checks and balances, their benevolent schemes on others. Some want to use that power to prevent suicide; others to provide suicide. Both groups insist that the practices they advocate constitute "medical care." I reject the definitions, assumptions, arguments, and tactics of the suicide preventers and suicide providers alike. Suicide is goal-directed behavior for which the actor has reasons and for which he, and he alone, is responsible. Medical considerations are as irrelevant to killing oneself as they are to killing others.

Our True Last Will: The Fatal Freedom

When we call the last testament the "last will," we are using a figure of speech. Our legal last will is usually prepared and executed long before we die. Our truly last will is the decision to kill ourselves, assuming that is how we want to die. Planning for suicide is an aspect of preparing for death, similar to preparing a health proxy or a last will.

As noted earlier, virtually every difficult decision we make—from choosing a career to choosing a mate—we must make too soon lest we make it too late and forfeit the chance to make it at all. The decision to kill oneself falls in that class. However, that does not justify our prohibiting people from making such a decision.

Allowing people to plan to end their lives would have the same consequences as does allowing them to plan to dispose of their property. The opportunity to plan for the future of one's property after one's life ends encourages individuals to be prudent about how they, not others or the State, see fit. Similarly, the opportunity to plan for the manner of one's death would encourage individuals to be prudent about how they live and would enable them to end their lives as they, not others or the State, choose.

What would be the consequences of a pragmatic-permissive attitude toward death control? Absent suicide prohibition (and drug prohibition), people would feel secure about having access to an emergency cord they could pull when they want to exit life, without interference by others. As a result, some people who now kill themselves too early lest they lose the chance to do so might postpone ending their lives and die of different causes; others, now deterred by drug and suicide prohibitions, might kill themselves once the impediments are removed. It is impossible to predict with certainty whether the right to practice death control would result in fewer or more suicides. Unless we prefer illusory security to true liberty, the result of abolishing antisuicide measures ought not influence our judgment about the legitimacy of a right to death control.

We can make decisions about birth control—whether it is right or wrong, whether to practice or forgo it—without help or hindrance by the State. Not until we can make decisions about death control without help or hindrance by the State will we be in formal possession of our most basic freedom: the freedom to decide when and how we die.

Appendix

The contemporary eye sees suicide either as an illness requiring medical measures to cope with it or as a treatment for the terminally ill requiring medical assistance with it. As a counterweight against that monochromatically distorted vision of voluntary death, in this Appendix I offer some different perceptions of and attitudes toward suicide.

TOLERATING SUICIDE: THOMAS JEFFERSON (1743–1826)

In 1779, the Virginia Legislature was considering a bill to repeal the punishment of suicide by the "forfeiture of chattels." Jefferson offered the following statement in its support:

Suicide is by law punishable by forfeiture of chattels. This bill [revising the Virginia code] exempts it from forfeiture. The suicide injures the State less than he who leaves it with his effects. If the latter then not be punished, the former should not. As to the example, we need not fear its influence. Men are too much attached to life, to exhibit frequent instances of depriving themselves of it. At any rate, the quasi-punishment of confiscation will not prevent it. For if one can be found who can calmly determine to renounce life, who is so weary of his existence here, as rather to make experiment of what is beyond the grave, can we suppose him, in such a state of mind, susceptible of influence from the losses to his family by confiscation? That men in general, too, disapprove of this severity, is apparent from the constant practice of juries finding the suicide in a state of insanity; because they have no other way of saving the forfeiture. Let it then be done away.[1]

On July 14, 1813, Jefferson replied to two letters he had received from Dr. Samuel Brown, who held the chair in the theory and practice of medicine at the University in Lexington, Virginia. The subject of their correspondence was, evidently, toxic plants useful for suicide, as in his response, Jefferson wrote:

The most elegant thing of that kind known is a preparation of the Jamestown weed, Datura-Stramonium, invented by the French in the time of Robespierre. Every man of firmness carried it constantly in his pocket to anticipate the guillotine. It brings on the deep sleep as quietly as fatigue does the ordinary sleep, without the least struggle or motion. . . . It seems far preferable to the Venesection of the Romans, the Hemlock of the Greeks, and the Opium of the Turks. . . . Could such a medicament be restrained to self-administration, it ought not to be kept secret. There are ills in life as desperate as intolerable, to which it would be the rational relief. . . . As a relief from tyranny indeed, for which the Romans recurred to it in the times of the emperors, it has been a wonder to me that they did not consider a poignard in the breast of the tyrant as a better remedy.[2]

DEFENDING SUICIDE: SIR LESLIE STEPHEN (1832–1904)

Leslie Stephen—the father of Virginia Woolf and the younger brother of James Fitjzames Stephen—was a prominent Victorian man of letters, deeply attached not only to reason and literature, but to atheism as well. His views and writings on suicide may have provided a moral rationale for Virginia's aggressive assertion of her right to kill herself. In 1882, in *The Science of Ethics*—against the mainstream of official Victorian thought, yet in a form deeply characteristic of his age and class—Stephen presented a passionate argument for the morality of voluntary death. He wrote:

If, now, we suppose that a man, knowing that life meant for him nothing but agony, and that moreover his life could not serve others, and was only going to give useless pain to his attendants, and perhaps involve the sacrifice of health to his wife and children, should commit suicide, what ought we to think of him? He would, no doubt, be breaking the accepted moral code; but why should he not break it? . . . May we not say that he is acting on a superior moral principle, and that because he is clearly diminishing the sum of human misery? . . . The conduct may spring either from cowardice or from a loftier motive than the ordinary, and the merit of the action is therefore not determinable; but, assuming the loftier motive, I can see no ground for disapproving that action which flows from it.[3]

Leslie Stephen did not kill himself. He chose to die a painful and lingering death from cancer.

GLORIFYING SUICIDE: HENRY L. MENCKEN (1880–1956)

H. L. Mencken admired Friedrich Nietzsche (1844–1900) and was influenced by his writings. The excerpts that follow illustrate Nietzsche's and

Mencken's views on suicide. The contrast between the unpretentious and mocking style in which they wrote about voluntary death contrasts sharply with the pretentious and medicalized style in which modern journalists and opinion-makers write about it.

Death.—It is Schopenhauer's argument in his essay "On Suicide,"that the possibility of easy and painless self-destruction is the only thing that constantly and considerably ameliorates the horror of human life. Suicide is a means of escape from the world and its tortures—and therefore it is good. It is an ever-present refuge for the weak, the weary and the hopeless. . . . In all of this exaltation of surrender, of course, there is nothing whatever in common with the Dionysian philosophy of defiance. Nietzsche's teaching is all in the other direction. He urges, not surrender, but battle; not flight, but war to the end. His curse falls upon those "preachers of death" who counsel "an abandonment of life"—whether this abandonment be partial, as in asceticism, or actual, as in suicide. And yet Zarathustra sings the song of "free death" and says that the higher man must learn "to die at the right time." . . . Schopenhauer regards suicide as a means of escape, Nietzsche sees it as a means of good riddance. It is time to die, says Zarathustra, when the purpose of life ceases to be attainable—when the fighter breaks his sword arm or falls into his enemy's hands. And it is time to die, too, when the purpose of life is attained—when the fighter triumphs and sees before him no more worlds to conquer. . . . One who has "waxed too old for victories," one who is "yellow and wrinkled," one with a "toothless mouth"—for such an one a certain and speedy death. . . .

The best death is that which comes in battle "at the moment of victory"; the second best is death in battle in the hour of defeat. "Would that a storm came," sings Zarathustra, "to shake from the tree of life all those apples that are putrid and gnawed by worms. It is cowardice that maketh them stick to their branches"—cowardice which makes them afraid to die. But there is another cowardice which makes men afraid to live, and this is the cowardice of the Schopenhauerean pessimist. Nietzsche has no patience with it. To him a too early death seems as abominable as a death postponed too long. . . . Therefore Nietzsche pleads for an intelligent regulation of death. One must not die too soon and one must not die too late. "Natural death," he says, "is destitute of rationality. It is really irrational death, for the pitiable substance of the shell determines how long the kernel shall exist. The pining, sottish prison-warder decides the hour at which his noble prisoner is to die. . . . The enlightened regulation and control of death belongs to the morality of the future. At present religion makes it seem immoral, for religion presupposes that when the time for death comes, God gives the command."[4]

Nietzsche himself wrote: "There are states in which it is indecent to live any longer. . . . We must transform the stupid fact of physiology into a moral necessity. [Natural death] is death under the most contemptible circumstances, an unfree death, death at the wrong time, the death of a coward. From sheer love of life we should will death to be otherwise, free, conscious, without surprise, and non-accidental."[5] Sadly, Nietzsche's own protracted, pathetic death was just the sort of demise that he abhorred and denounced.

PROVOKING SUICIDE: LUDWIG II, KING OF BAVARIA (1845–1886)

Ludwig II became the ruler of Bavaria when he was nineteen, after the death of his father. He was a popular king. Unlike other royal wastrels, he did not indulge himself at the cost of public funds. He spent his own vast assets, mainly on building projects such as the construction of the famous castle at Neuschwanstein, today the principal tourist attraction in Bavaria. However, Ludwig was a homosexual at a time when homosexuality was considered to be a serious mental illness.

The independence of Bavaria stood in the way of Bismarck's efforts to create a united Germany. Bismarck was not only a political genius, he was also the first modern politician to perceive and make use of the possibilities of enlisting psychiatry directly in the service of the State: He knew how to play the insanity card long before playing it became an accepted judicial and political practice, in democratic and totalitarian countries alike. Unable to join Bavaria to Germany by diplomacy, Bismarck turned to psychiatry for help. In 1886, he proposed to Dr. Bernard van Gudden, professor of psychiatry at the University of Munich, that Ludwig be deposed by declaring him insane. Gudden jumped at the opportunity to demonstrate the usefulness of psychiatry to power. Although he had never met the king, he prepared a draft of his "medical findings," based on rumors about the "patient." To give his "findings" a veneer of authenticity, he "consulted" with three distinguished colleagues. Then, the four eminent psychiatrists signed a document in which they declared:

His Majesty is psychically disturbed in an advanced degree, suffering from the kind of mental sickness which psychiatrists know well and call paranoia (insanity). In view of this form of sickness and its gradual and progressive development over a great number of years, His Majesty must be declared incurable, for a further deterioration of his mental powers appears certain. Because of his sickness the exercise of His Majesty's free will is rendered completely impossible and His Majesty must be considered hindered in the exercise of government, which impediment will last not only longer than a year, but for his entire lifetime.[6]

After Ludwig was apprehended, the psychiatrists faced the problem of what to do with him. "Hospitalizing" the king in a private or a public insane asylum was out of the question. Instead, arrangements were made to place Ludwig under a kind of psychiatric house arrest: Berg Castle, one of the royal palaces situated by Lake Starnberg, was converted into an asylum, for the sole use of the royal patient. Recognizing that he had been sentenced to life imprisonment without any hope of parole, Ludwig decided to kill himself. On a pleasant day in June 1886, only two days after being installed at Berg Castle, the king and Dr. Gudden went for a walk by the lake. With the attendants guarding the king walking a polite distance behind them, Ludwig dashed into the lake. Gudden, much older and weaker than the youthful king, dashed after him. Before the guards could reach them, Ludwig drowned Gudden and then himself.[7]

RECOMMENDING SUICIDE: SIR WILLIAM OSLER (1849–1919)

A founder of the Johns Hopkins University Medical School and later Regius professor of medicine at Oxford, Osler was recognized as "the foremost spokesman for the medical profession throughout the English-speaking world."[8] In 1905, the year he left Baltimore for Oxford, he delivered a public address, titled "The Fixed Period," in which he declared that men over the age of sixty were useless and that "peaceful departure by chloroform might lead to incalculable benefits," for them as well as for society.[9] Osler later said, not very persuasively, that his proposal was "whimsical." However, many people took it seriously. His supposed spoof had temporarily enriched the language, generating the verb "to Oslerize," used both in jest and in earnest.

When Osler delivered his speech on suicide, he was a revered figure in American medicine. Nevertheless, the press—then still vigilant about protecting personal freedom from medical statism—was alarmed. An editorial in the *New York Times* castigated his remarks and compared his proposal to the practices of "savage tribes . . . whose custom it is to knock their elders on the head whenever the juniors find their elders in their own way."[10] Two days after the address was denounced in the papers, a Civil War veteran shot himself to death. A clipping of Osler's address was found on his desk. The story was front-page news in a report entitled "Suicide Had Osler Speech." Undaunted, Osler angrily retorted: "I meant just what I said, but it's disgraceful, this fuss that the newspapers are making about it." In his hagiography of Osler, Harvey Cushing, the famed Harvard neurosurgeon, stated: "Efforts were made in vain to get him to refute his statement; and though there can be no question that he was sorely hurt, he went on his way with a smile."[11]

The occasion for Osler's famous "chloroform address" was his resignation from Hopkins to accept the position of Regius professor of medicine at Oxford. Nearly fifty-six years old, he was contemplating his own aging. In his speech, Osler asserted that "men above sixty years of age [are] useless," and concluded "that the history of the world shows that a very large proportion of the evils may be traced to sexagenarians—nearly all the great mistakes politically and socially."[12] The view that Osler was serious is supported by his favorable reference to John Donne's *Biathanatos*[13] and to the fact that his essay was partly inspired by Anthony Trollope's (1815–1882) *The Fixed Period.* That story, cast in the familiar mold of a futuristic utopia/dystopia, takes place on the imaginary island, "Britanulla," where the human life span is fixed at sixty-five years.[14] At the end of their sixty-sixth year, men and women are admitted to a college for a twelve-month period of preparation for euthanasia by chloroform. Trollope was sixty-seven when he wrote the novel. He died a year later, without benefit of chloroform.

Despite his stature as the giant of American medicine, Osler never lived down his flirting with medical killing. Prior to World War I, Americans still ranked personal self-reliance more highly than statist protectionism and recognized that Osler, regardless of his professional qualifications, was a medical socialist, on the model of Otto Bismarck. Osler admired German medical statism, especially its alleged advances in understanding "insanity." He was instrumental in adding psychiatry to the medical curriculum at Hopkins by persuading his friend, the philanthropist Henry Phipps, to underwrite the founding of what became the Phipps Psychiatric Clinic.[15]

Notes

PREFACE

1. J. S. Mill, *On Liberty*, p. 52.
2. T. S. Szasz, *The Second Sin*, p. 76.
3. A. Camus, *The Myth of Sisyphus*, p. 1.

CHAPTER 1 SPEAKING OF SUICIDE

1. St. Augustine, quoted in G. Rosen, "History in the Study of Suicide," *Psychological Medicine* 1 (1971): 270.
2. "Banishing Books?" *U.S. News & World Report*, 18 May 1992, p. 76.
3. E. Gibbon, *The Decline and Fall of the Roman Empire*, p. 232.
4. D. Daube, "The Linguistics of Suicide," *Philosophy and Public Affairs* 1 (1972): 390.
5. Ibid., p. 415.
6. Ibid., pp. 394, 393.
7. B. Barraclough and D. Shepherd, "A Necessary Neologism: The Origin and Uses of Suicide," *Suicide and Life-Threatening Behavior* 24 (Summer 1994): 118.
8. W. W. Westcott, *Suicide*, p. 31.
9. T. S. Szasz, *The Meaning of Mind*, pp. 105–8.
10. M. Taylor and H. Ryan, "Fanaticism, Political Suicide, and Terrorism," *Terrorism* 11 (1988): 91–111.
11. See for example, Associated Press, "Extremists Line up to Be Suicide Bombers in Germany," *Syracuse Herald-Journal*, 18 April 1997, p. A1.
12. See M. McLuhan, *The Gutenberg Galaxy*; and also, J. C. Carson, "Culture, Psychiatry, and the Written Word," *Psychiatry* 22 (November 1959): 307–20.
13. T. Aquinas, *The Summa Theologica*, p. 209.

14. T. S. Szasz, "The Illusion of Mental Patients' Rights," in T. S. Szasz, *A Lexicon of Lunacy*, pp. 127–41; especially pp. 134–35.

15. F. J. Cornell, "Double Effect, Principle of," in *New Catholic Encyclopedia*, vol. 4, pp. 1020–22.

16. D. H. Smith, "On Paul Ramsey: A Covenant-Centered Ethic for Medicine," *Second Opinion* 6 (November 1987): 108; emphasis added.

17. M. Taylor and H. Ryan, "Fanaticism, Political Suicide, and Terrorism," *Terrorism* 11 (1988): 91.

CHAPTER 2 CONSTRUCTING SUICIDE

1. D. Hume, "Essay I," in D. Hume, *Essays on Suicide*, pp. 20–21.

2. J.E.D. Esquirol, *Mental Maladies*, p. 307.

3. R.J.Z. Werblowsky and G. Wigoder, eds., *The Encyclopedia of the Jewish Religion*, p. 367.

4. A.J.L. van Hooff, *From Autothanasia to Suicide*, p. 141.

5. Plato, *Phaedo*, trans. by Hugh Tredennick, 61 c–e, in *The Collected Dialogues of Plato*, p. 44.

6. Ibid., 62 b–c, p. 45.

7. Ibid., 62 c, 80 b, 107 c, pp. 45, 63, 89.

8. E. Hamilton and H. Cairns, in ibid., p. 40.

9. Plato, *Laws*, 873 c–d, in ibid., p. 1432.

10. Aristotle, *Ethica Nicomachea* (Nicomachean Ethics), 1138a, in *The Basic Works of Aristotle*, p. 1021.

11. A.J.L. van Hoof, *From Autothanasia to Suicide*, p. 122.

12. See p. 16.

13. A.J.L. van Hoof, *From Autothanasia to Suicide*, pp. 41, 123–24.

14. Quoted in ibid., p. 190.

15. 1 Samuel 31:4.

16. Judges 16:28–30.

17. Matthew 27:1–5.

18. Quoted in G. Rosen, "History in the Study of Suicide," *Psychological Medicine* 1 (1971): 270.

19. E. Gibbon, *The Decline and Fall of the Roman Empire*, p. 327.

20. A.J.L. van Hooff, *From Autothanasia to Suicide*, p. 273; and A. J. Droge and J. D. Tabor, *A Noble Death*, p. 6.

21. G. M. Carstairs, quoted in in E. Stengel, *Suicide*, p. 7.

22. R.J.Z. Werblowsky and G. Wigoder, eds., *The Encyclopedia of the Jewish Religion*, p. 367. See also, J. Goldin, ed., *The Living Talmud*.

23. "Catholic Church Says It Won't 'Judge' White," *San Francisco Chronicle*, 22 October 1983, p. 3.

24. S. E. Sprott, *The English Debate on Suicide*, p. 157.

25. M. Macdonald, "Suicidal Behaviour: Social Section," in G. E. Berrios and R. Porter, eds., *A History of Clinical Psychiatry*, p. 626.

26. D. Erasmus, *In Praise of Folly*, p. 60, quoted in G. Rosen, "History in the Study of Suicide," *Psychological Medicine* 1 (1971): 275.

27. Quoted in G. Rosen, "History in the Study of Suicide," *Psychological Medicine* 1 (1971): 275.

28. Montesquieu, quoted in ibid., p. 279.

29. J. Donne, *Biathanatos*, p. 18.

30. Ibid., pp. 11, 13–14.

31. See generally, G. Williams, "Suicide," in *Encyclopedia of Philosophy*, vol. 8, pp. 43–46.

32. I. Kant, "Suicide," in S. Gorowitz et al., eds., *Moral Problems in Medicine*, pp. 377–381.

33. T. S. Szasz, *Cruel Compassion*, Chapter 6.

34. L. M. Cohen, "Suicide, Hastening Death, and Psychiatry," *Archives of Internal Medicine* 158 (12 October 1998): 1973.

35. M. Macdonald, "Suicidal Behaviour: Social Section," in G. E. Berrios and R. Porter, eds., *A History of Clinical Psychiatry*, pp. 627, 630.

36. J.E.D. Esquirol, quoted in G. Rosen, "History in the Study of Suicide," *Psychological Medicine* 1 (1971): 281; and J.E.D. Esquirol, *Mental Maladies*, p. 21.

37. E. Kraepelin, *Lectures on Clinical Psychiatry*, pp. 2–3, 9.

38. Quoted in J. D. Droge and A. J. Tabor, *A Noble Death*, p. 6.

39. Associated Press, "Killer Who Took Overdose Is Revived, Then Executed," *Syracuse Herald Journal*, 11 August 1995, p. A9.

40. E. Stengel, *Suicide*, p. 71.

41. L. M. Cohen, "Suicide, Hastening Death, and Psychiatry," *Archives of Internal Medicine* 158 (12 October 1998): 1973.

42. E. Stengel, *Suicide*, p. 71.

43. J. Motto, "Commentaries," in M. P. Battin and A. G. Lipman, eds., *Drug Use in Assisted Suicide and Euthanasia*, p. 307.

44. S. Freud, "Contributions to a Discussion on Suicide" (1910), in SE [*Standard Edition*], vol. 11, p. 232.

45. S. Freud, "Mourning and Melancholia" (1917), SE, vol. 14, p. 252. See also, "The Psychogenesis of a Case of Homosexuality in a Woman" (1920), SE, vol. 18, p. 162.

46. R. Noll, *The Aryan Christ*, p. 151.

47. C. G. Jung, "Letter to Anonymous," 13 October 1951, in *C. G. Jung Letters*, vol. 2, p. 25.

48. I. Veith, "Reflections on the Medical History of Suicide," *Modern Medicine*, 11 August 1969, p. 116.

49. "Changing Concepts of Suicide" (Editorial), *Journal of the American Medical Association* 199 (March 1967): 162.

50. S. Yolles, "The Tragedy of Suicide in the United States," in L. Yochelson, ed., *Symposium on Suicide*, pp. 16–17.

51. H. Hendin and G. Klerman, "Physician-Assisted Suicide: The Dangers of Legalization," *American Journal of Psychiatry* 150 (January 1993): 143–45.

52. E. Shneidman, "Suicide," in *Encyclopedia Britannica*, vol. 21, p. 384.

53. American Association of Suicidology, "Understanding and Preventing Suicide" (Washington, DC: pamphlet, n.d.).

54. N. St. John-Stevas, *Life, Death, and the Law*, p. 243. For a comprehensive review see, T. J. Marzen et al., "Suicide: A Constitutional Right?" *Duquesne Law Review* 1 (Fall 1985): 1–241.

55. *Donaldson v. Van De Kamp*, 4 Cal. Rptr. 2d 59 (Cal. App. 2 Dist. 1992), p. 64.

56. S. Perlin, "Legal Aspects of Suicide," in L. D. Hankoff and B. Einsidler, eds., *Suicide*, p. 93.

57. Quoted in L. Greenhouse, "High Court Hears 2 Cases Involving Assisted Suicide," *New York Times*, 9 January 1997, pp. A1, B9; and A. Lewis, "Perchance to Dream," *New York Times*, 10 January 1997, p. A33.

58. C. K. Smith, "Current Law on Physician-Assisted Suicide for the Terminally Ill," in M. P. Battin and A. G. Lipman, eds., *Drug Use in Assisted Suicide and Euthanasia*, p. 141.

59. A. G. McCoy, "HIV Disease: Criminal and Civil Liability for Assisted Suicide," *Golden Gate University Law Review* 21 (1991): 440.

60. For further discussion, see chapter 6.

61. T. S. Szasz, *Our Right to Drugs*, Chapter 3.

62. E. Kriss, "Lecturer Claims Rock Music Is Catalyst for Teen Suicide," *Syracuse Herald-Journal*, 19 November 1984, p. B1; United Press International, "Expert: Rock Music a Factor in Suicides," *Syracuse Post-Standard*, 27 October 1984, p. A2; J. Pareles, "Too Heavy? Some Parents, Lawyers Charge Song's Lyrics Can Kill," *Syracuse Herald-Journal*, 27 October 1988, pp. D1, D16.

63. A. G. McCoy, "HIV Disease: Criminal and Civil Liability for Assisted Suicide," *Golden Gate University Law Review* 21 (1991): 443.

64. D. Stout, "A Hearing Focuses on Lyrics Laced with Violence and Death," *New York Times*, 7 November 1997, p. A21. See also, *McCollum v. CBS, Inc.*, 249 Cal. Rptr. 187 (Cal. App. 2 Dist. 1988).

65. "Looking Forward to Trip Going to the Next Level," *New York Times*, 28 March 1997, p. A19.

66. R. Hampson, "Monk Saw Martyrdom, Embraced Own Death," *Syracuse Herald-American*, 30 March 1997, p. C1; and "The Testament of Dom Christian de Cherge" (1993), *Syracuse Herald-American*, 30 March 1997, p. C1.

67. For a striking example, see C. Goldberg, "After Suicide, Harvard Alters Policies on Graduate Students," *New York Times*, 21 October, 1998, p. A20.

68. P. Manso, "Chronicle of a Tragedy Foretold," *The New York Times Magazine*, 19 July 1998, pp. 32–37.

69. Quoted in E. Duggan, "Fall's Cause Unclear," *Syracuse Herald-Journal*, 29 June 1998, p. B1; E. Duggan, "Cold Tablet 'High' Proved Fatal for Teen Who Jumped at Mall," *Syracuse Herald-American*, 19 July 1998, pp. A1, A6.

70. M. Simons, "Serb Charged with Massacre Commits Suicide," *New York Times*, 30 June 1998, p. A6; Associated Press, "Serb Awaiting Verdict Commits Suicide," *Syracuse Herald-Journal*, 30 June 1998, p. A3.

71. A. Toufexis, "Warnings about a Miracle Drug: Reports of Suicide Attempts in Prozac Users Raise Doubts about the Popular Antidepressant," *Time*, 30 July 1990, p. 54; N. Angier, "Suicidal Behavior Tied Again to Drug," *New York Times*, 7 February 1991, p. B15.

72. See J. Cornwell, *The Power to Harm*.

73. Cicero, quoted in N. Guterman, ed., *The Anchor Book of Latin Quotations*, pp. 52–53.

74. Quoted in J. H. Newton, "Are Clinton's Aides so Innocent?" (Letter to the Editor), *New York Times*, 22 September 1998, p. A30.

75. P. J. Boyer, "Life after Vince," *The New Yorker*, 11 September 1995, pp. 54–67.

CHAPTER 3 EXCUSING SUICIDE

1. J. F. Stephen, *A History of the Criminal Law of England*, vol. 2, p. 185.

2. H. G. Wells, *Love and Mrs. Lewisham*, p. 205.

3. J. Goebbels, quoted in M. Heller, *Cogs in the Wheel*, p. 233.

4. R. Burton, *The Anatomy of Melancholy*.

5. R. Burton, quoted in G. Rosen, "History in the Study of Suicide," *Psychological Medicine* 1 (1971): 275–76; emphasis added.

6. R. Burton, quoted in R. Hunter and I. Macalpine, *Three Hundred Years of Psychiatry*, p. 95.

7. R. Burton, *The Anatomy of Melancholy*, pp. 224–26.

8. T. S. Szasz, *Law, Liberty, and Psychiatry*, and *Insanity*, pp. 138–40.

9. J. Sym, quoted in R. Hunter and I. Macalpine, *Three Hundred Years of Psychiatry*, pp. 113, 114–15.

10. G. Harvey, quoted in ibid., pp. 196–97.

11. G. Cheyne, *The English Malady*, p. 111.

12. See generally, W. L. Parry-Jones, *The Trade in Lunacy*.

13. T. S. Szasz, *Insanity*, and *Cruel Compassion*.

14. W. Blackstone, *Commentaries on the Laws of England*, pp. 211–12.

15. Ibid., p. 212.

16. S. E. Sprott, *The English Debate on Suicide*, p. 112; emphasis added.

17. "Londonderry, Robert Stewart," in *Encyclopaedia Britannica*, vol. 14, pp. 291–93; and M. Macdonald, "Suicidal Behavior," in G. Berrios and R. Porter, eds., *A History of Clinical Psychiatry*, p. 630.

18. T. S. Szasz, *Law, Liberty, and Psychiatry*, p. 212.

19. H. C. Black, *Black's Law Dictionary*, p. 881.

20. T. S. Szasz, *Psychiatric Justice*.

21. For a more detailed discussion, see T. S. Szasz, *Insanity*.

22. R. Maudsley, *Responsibility in Mental Disease*, pp. 123, 133; emphasis added.

23. Ibid., pp. 136–37; emphasis added.

24. K. Menninger, *The Crime of Punishment*, p. 265.

25. T. Borge, quoted in T. G. Ash, "God and the Revolution," *Spectator* (London), 24 March 1984, p. 8.

26. *M'Naghten's Case*, 10 Cl. & F. 200, 8 Eng. Rep. 718 (H.L.), 1843. See generally, R. Smith, *Trial by Medicine*.

27. *M'Naghten's Case*, 10 Cl. & F. 200, 8 Eng. Rep. 718 (H.L.), 1843; *The Queen Against Daniel McNaghten*, 1843, Central Criminal Court, Old Bailey, in D. J. West and A. Walk, eds., *Daniel McNaghten*, pp. 12–13. Subsequent references are to this source.

28. Ibid., pp. 22, 29.

29. R. Smith, *Trial by Medicine*, p. 103.

30. *The Queen Against Daniel McNaghten*, in D. J. West and A. Walk, eds., *Daniel McNaghten*, p. 72; emphasis added.

31. Ibid., p. 73.

32. Ibid., p. 31.

33. R. Smith, *Trial by Medicine*, p. 23.

34. H. Maudsley, *Responsibility in Mental Disease*, pp. 15, 42, 163, 198.

35. J. F. Stephen, *A History of the Criminal Law of England*, vol. 2, pp. 128, 131–32.

36. Ibid., p. 130.

37. Ibid., p. 177; emphasis added.

38. Ibid., p. 181.

39. Ibid., pp. 179, 185.

40. Ibid., p. 107.

41. G. B. Chisholm, "The Psychiatry of Enduring Peace and Social Progress," *Psychiatry* (1946): 9.

42. K. Menninger, *The Vital Balance*, pp. 32–33.

43. K. Menninger, *The Crime of Punishment*, p. 265.

CHAPTER 4 "PREVENTING" SUICIDE

1. E. Bleuler, *Dementia Praecox*, pp. 488–89; emphasis added.

2. A. J. Prange, Jr., "Antidepressants," in S. Arieti, ed., *American Handbook of Psychiatry*, 2nd ed., vol. 5, pp. 476–77.

3. E. Shneidman, *The Suicidal Mind*, p. 166.

4. D. Schaffer, "Suicide: Risk Factors and the Public Health" (Editorial), *American Journal of Public Health* 83 (February 1993): 171–72. The author is a child psychiatrist.

5. T. S. Szasz, "The Ethics of Suicide," *The Antioch Review* 31 (Spring 1971): 7–17; reprinted in T. S. Szasz, *The Theology of Medicine*, pp. 68–85.

6. S. Stamberg, quoted in C. Hitchens, "Smoke and Mirrors," *Vanity Fair*, October 1994, p. 95.

7. Cited in T. S. Szasz, *The Theology of Medicine*, p. 83; emphasis added.

8. Cited in ibid., p. 82; emphasis added.

9. J. Stage, "Two Officers Talk Man from Jumping off Bridge: They Said They Worked to Establish Rapport with Him," *Syracuse Herald-Journal*, 27 December 1997, p. A4; emphasis added.

10. Associated Press, "Woman's Body Found," *Syracuse Herald-Journal*, 26 March 1997, p. A12.

11. H. C. Black, *Black's Law Dictionary*, pp. 1352, 1358.

12. M. Newman, "A Fight to Acknowledge a Life: Mother's Efforts Help Alter Policy on Suicide Victims," *New York Times*, 24 February 1998, pp. B1, B4.

13. R. Neugebauer, "Diagnosis, Guardianship, and Residential Care of the Mentally Ill in Medieval and Early Modern England," *American Journal of Psychiatry* 146 (December 1989): 1580; emphasis added.

14. Ibid., p. 1582.

15. S. Tuke, *Description of the Retreat*, p. 144.

16. Ibid., pp. 163–87.

17. A. Digby, "Moral Treatment at the Retreat, 1796–1846," in W. F. Bynum, R. Porter, and M. Shepherd, eds., *The Anatomy of Madness*, vol. 2, p. 60.

18. T. S. Szasz, "Noncoercive Psychiatry: An Oxymoron," *Journal of Humanistic Psychology* 31 (Spring 1991): 117–25.

19. A. Roy, "Preface," in A. Roy, ed., *Suicide*, p. vii.

20. E. Shneidman, "Preventing Suicide," *Bulletin of Suicidology* 20 (1968): 1.

21. E. Stengel, *Suicide*, p. 143.

22. E. Shneidman, *The Suicidal Mind*.

23. Ibid., pp. 4–5, 160.

24. Ibid., p. 161; emphasis added.

25. Ibid., p. 165.

26. Ibid., p. 166.

27. R. W. Firestone, *Suicide and the Inner Voice*, p. 61.

28. Ibid., pp. 118, 248; emphasis added.

29. J. B. Robitscher, *The Powers of Psychiatry*, p. 130.

30. A. M. Jeger, "Behavior Theories and Their Application," in L. D. Hankoff and B. Einsidler, eds., *Suicide*, p. 196; see also I. Trowell, "Telephone Services," in ibid., pp. 401–9.

31. Research and Clinical News, "Suicide Rates Have not Fallen Despite Better Psychotropics," *Psychiatric News*, 16 January 1998.

32. E. Stengel, *Suicide*, p. 13.

33. A. Artaud, "Van Gogh, the Man Suicided by Society" (1947), in A. Artaud, *Selected Writings*, pp. 496–97.

34. L. D. Hankoff and B. Einsidler, "The Dialectics of Suicide," in L. D. Hankoff and B. Einsidler, eds., *Suicide*, pp. 415–16.

35. P. Solomon, "The Burden of Responsibility in Suicide," *JAMA* 199 (January 1967): 324.

36. I. Berlin, "My Intellectual Path" (1996), *New York Review of Books*, 14 May 1998, pp. 58–59.

37. *Nally v. Grace Community Church*, 47 Cal. 3d 278 (1988), p. 98; emphasis added.

38. W. Freeman, "Psychosurgery," in S. Arieti, ed., *American Handbook of Psychiatry*, vol. 2, p. 1527.

39. A. J. Prange, Jr., "Antidepressants," in S. Arieti, ed., *American Handbook of Psychiatry*, 2nd ed., vol. 5, pp. 476–77.

40. T. Jefferson, "Notes on Religion" (1776), in T. Jefferson, *Thomas Jefferson on Democracy*, p. 109.

41. T. S. Szasz, "The Political Legitimation of Quackery," *Reason* 29 (March 1998): 25–26.

42. E. Thomas et al., "A Matter of Honor," *Newsweek*, 27 May 1996, pp. 24–29.

43. D. Stout, "Trapped, Fugitive Ex-prosecutor Kills Himself in Nevada Hotel," *New York Times*, 27 November 1996, p. B5; W. Glaberson, "Depressed, Bissell Fled without Plan, Lawyer Says," *New York Times*, 30 November 1996, p. 30; W.

Glaberson, "In Prosecutor's Rise and Fall, a Story of Ambition, Deceit and Shame," *New York Times*, 1 December 1996, p. 52.

44. "Student Kills Counselor Who Reported Drug Use," *Syracuse Herald-Journal*, 7 October 1996, p. A6.

45. "Suicide Victim Mistakenly Feared '3-Strikes' Fate," *Syracuse Herald-Journal*, 7 October 1996, p. A6.

46. M. Swartz, "Family Secret," *The New Yorker*, 17 November 1997, p. 90.

47. S. Rimer, "Killer of Two Abortion Clinic Workers Is Found Dead of Asphyxiation in Prison Cell," *New York Times*, 30 November 1996, p. 9.

48. M. Swartz, "Family Secret," *The New Yorker*, 17 November 1997, p. 107.

49. R. E. Schulman, "Suicide and Suicide Prevention: A Legal Analysis," *American Bar Association Journal* 54 (September 1968): 862.

50. See *Natanson v. Kline*, 186 Kan. 393, 404, P. 2d 1093, p. 1104 (1960); and *In re Estate of Brooks*, 205 N.E. 2d 435 (Ill. 1965).

51. A. Roy, "Suicide in Doctors," *Psychiatric Clinics of North America* 8 (June 1985): 377–87.

52. P. A. Boxer, C. Burnett, and N. Swanson, "Suicide and Occupation: A Review of the Literature," *Journal of Occupational and Environmental Medicine* 37 (April 1995): 442, 445.

53. L. Krieger, "Preventing Physician Suicides," *American Medical News*, 5 May 1985, pp. 3, 21.

54. "Suicide-Prevention Program to Be Explored by Board," *American Medical News*, 27 June–4 July 1996, p. 30.

CHAPTER 5 PRESCRIBING SUICIDE

1. G. Williams, "Mercy-Killing Legislation: A Rejoinder," in T. Beauchamp and L. Walters, eds., *Contemporary Issues in Bioethics*, p. 323.

2. Quoted in R. Dworkin et al., "Assisted Suicide: The Philosophers' Brief," *New York Review of Books*, 27 March 1997, p. 45.

3. D. Bonhoeffer, *Ethics*, p. 162; emphasis added.

4. A.J.L. van Hooff, *From Autothanasia to Suicide*, p. 51.

5. T. More, *Utopia*, p. 18.

6. Quoted in E. J. Emanuel, "The History of Euthanasia Debates in the United States and Britain," *Annals of Internal Medicine* 121 (15 November 1994): 793–94.

7. J. C. Warren, *Etherization*, p. 33.

8. E. J. Emanuel, "The History of Euthanasia Debates in the United States and Britain," *Annals of Internal Medicine* 121 (15 November 1994): 794. In this connection, see W. Osler, "The Fixed Period," in W. Osler, *Aequanimitas*, pp. 375–93; and H. A. Johnson, "Osler Recommends Chloroform at Sixty," *The Pharos* 59 (Winter 1996): 24–26.

9. For a review of the legal literature, see C. DeSimone, *Death on Demand*.

10. B. Keizer, *Dancing with Mr. D*.

11. J. F. Stephen, *A History of the Criminal Law of England*, vol. 2, p. 230.

12. H. C. Black, *Black's Law Dictionary*, pp. 29–30.

13. R. Kennedy, "Doctor Is Arraigned in Assisted Suicide," *New York Times*, 15 October 1998, p. B3.

14. G. Kolata, "Documents Like Living Wills Are Rarely of Aid, Study Says," *New York Times*, 8 April 1997, p. A12.

15. M. Clements and D. Hales, "In a New National Survey, Parade Asked: How Healthy Are We?" *Parade*, 7 September 1997, p. 4. See also, P. Wilkes, "The Next Pro-Lifers," *The New York Times Magazine*, 21 July 1996, p. 22 *ff*.

16. T. S. Szasz, *Our Right to Drugs*, pp. 125–43.

17. *Code of Federal Regulations*, 21 CFR 1306.04 (1996); emphasis added. See also, G. J. Annas, "Death by Prescription: The Oregon Initiative," *New England Journal of Medicine* 331 (3 November 1994): 1240–43.

18. T. S. Szasz, "The Fatal Temptation: Drug Prohibition and the Fear of Autonomy," *Daedalus* 121 (Summer 1992): 161–64.

19. *M'Naghten's Case*, 10 Cl. & F. 200, 8 Eng. Rep. 718 (H.L.), 1843; *The Queen Against Daniel McNaghten*, 1843, Central Criminal Court, Old Bailey, in D. J. West and A. Walk, eds., *Daniel McNaghten*, pp. 12–73.

20. *Roe v. Wade*, 410 U.S. 113, 93 S. Ct 705, 35 L. Ed.2d (1973).

21. *Compassion in Dying v. State of Wash.*, 79 F.3d 790 (9th Cir. 1996).

22. Quoted in W. J. Smith, "Death March," *National Review*, 23 February 1998, p. 34; emphasis added.

23. *Quill v. Vacco*, 80 F.3d 716 (2nd Cir. 1996), 721.

24. *Compassion in Dying v. State of Wash.*, 79 F.3d 790 (9th Cir. 1996), p. 791.

25. Ibid., p. 801.

26. "Bone Marrow Transplant in Fetus Staves off Immune Disease," *New York Times*, 12 December 1996, p. A27.

27. S. B. Donnelly, "The Postpartum Prosecutor," *Time*, 15 December 1997, p. 4.

28. *Compassion in Dying v. State of Wash.*, 79 F.3d 790 (9th Cir. 1996), p. 820; emphasis added.

29. Ibid., p. 834.

30. A. Alpers and B. Lo, "Physician-Assisted Suicide in Oregon: A Bold Experiment," *JAMA* 274 (9 August 1995): 483–87; emphasis added.

31. L. Greenhouse, "Court, 9–0, Upholds State Laws Prohibiting Assisted Suicide: No Help for Dying," *New York Times*, 27 June 1997, pp. A1, A19; J. Scott, "An Issue That Won't Die," *New York Times*, 27 June 1997, p. A1, A19; *Washington et al. v. Glucksberg*, 1997 WL. 348094; and *Vacco v. Quill*, 1997 WL. 348037.

32. W. H. Rehnquist, quoted in L. Greenhouse, "Court, 9–0, Upholds State Laws Prohibiting Assisted Suicide: No Help for Dying," *New York Times*, 27 June 1997, p. A1.

33. See chapter 1.

34. T. E. Quill, "Death and Dignity: A Case of Individualized Decision Making," *New England Journal of Medicine* 324 (March 1991): 693; T. E. Quill, B. Lo, and D. W. Brock, "Palliative Options of Last Resort: A Comparison of Voluntarily Stopping Eating and Drinking, Terminal Sedation, Physician-Assisted Suicide, and Voluntary Active Euthanasia," *JAMA* 278 (17 December 1997): 2100; T. E.

Quill, *Death and Dignity*, p. 164; and *Compassion in Dying v. State of Wash.*, 79 F.3d 790 (9th Cir. 1996), p. 811.

35. *Compassion in Dying v. State of Wash.*, 79 F.3d 790 (9th Cir. 1996), p. 823; emphasis added.

36. Ibid., p. 824.

37. Ibid.; emphasis added.

38. "1995 Oregon Laws," Chapter 3, p. 666; also cited in A. Alpers and B. Lo, "Physician-Assisted Suicide in Oregon: A Bold Experiment," *JAMA* 274 (9 August 1995): 484.

39. P. R. Muskin, "Legislating Suicide" (Letter to the Editor), *New York Times*, 23 September 1998, p. A28; emphasis added.

40. T. S. Szasz, "Bootlegging Humanistic Values Through Psychiatry," *Antioch Review* 22 (Fall 1962): 341–49; reprinted in T. S. Szasz, *Ideology and Insanity*, pp. 87–97; and T. S. Szasz, "The Ethics of Abortion," *Humanist* 26 (September–October 1966): 147–48.

41. P. V. Admiraal, "Euthanasia in the Netherlands," *Free Inquiry* 17 (Winter 1996-97): 7.

42. See chapter 7.

43. R. Daly, "May Physicians Cause Death?" *Alumni Journal*, SUNY Health Science Center, Syracuse (Winter 1997): 34–35.

44. Ibid.

45. W. Shakespeare, *The Winter's Tale*, I, i, 18.

46. See generally T. S. Szasz, *The Manufacture of Madness*.

47. For an exception, see M. Betzold, "The Selling of Doctor Death," *New Republic*, 26 May 1997, pp. 22–26.

48. J. Kevorkian, *Prescription*, p. 202.

49. Ibid., p. 203.

50. Ibid., pp. 233–35; emphasis added.

51. Ibid., p. 217; emphasis added.

52. Ibid., p. 141.

53. Ibid., pp. 184, 158; emphasis added.

54. Ibid., pp. 195–200.

55. Ibid., p. 200; emphasis added.

56. M. Williams, *Cry of Pain*, p. 105. Williams mistakenly identifies Derek Humphry the same way.

57. B. Harmon, "The Many Faces of Jack Kevorkian," *Detroit News*, 23 February 1997, pp. 1A, 8A.

58. Associated Press, "Kevorkian Says He Helps to Relieve Pain, Suffering," *Syracuse Herald-Journal*, 2 March 1996, p. A2.

59. Quoted in J. Lessenberry, "Kevorkian Indicted on Charges of Helping in Three Suicides," *New York Times*, 1 November 1996, p. A32; B. Varner, "Kevorkian vs. the Prosecutor," *USA Today*, 1 November 1996, p. 3A; and J. Lessenberry, "Kevorkian Is Arrested and Charged in Suicide," *New York Times*, 8 November, 1996, p. A19.

60. J. Kevorkian, *Prescription*, p. 184.

61. D. Goodman, "Kevorkian: Kidneys not Likely to Be Used," *Syracuse Herald-Journal*, 8 June 1998, p. A1; M. Lasalandra, "Kidney Offer Criticized: Transplant Experts Say Kevorkian Plan an Outrage," *Boston Herald*, 9 June 1998, p. A4.

62. C. S. Lewis, "The Humanitarian Theory of Punishment" (1953), in C. S. Lewis, *God in the Dock*, p. 293.

63. *Quill v. Vacco*, 80 F.3d 716 (2nd Cir.) 1996, p. 721.

64. Quoted in L. Montgomery, "Death's Other Image: By Name, Face, or Method, He's No Jack Kevorkian," *Free Press* (Detroit), 16 December 1996, pp. 1A, 6A.

65. Ibid.

66. T. E. Quill, *A Midwife Through the Dying Process*, p. 4.

67. Ibid., p. 202.

68. Ibid.; emphasis added.

69. Ibid., p. 198.

70. Ibid., pp. 81, 82.

71. Ibid., p. 89.

72. Ibid.

73. Ibid., p. 202.

74. T. E. Quill, quoted in L. Montgomery, "Death's Other Image: By Name, Face, or Method, He's No Jack Kevorkian," *Free Press* (Detroit), 16 December 1996, pp. 1A, 6A.

75. T. E. Quill, quoted in L. Reibstein and D. Klaidman, "Weighing the Right to Die," *Newsweek*, 13 January 1997, p. 62.

76. J. Madison, quoted in S. Moore, "Our Unconstitutional Congress," *Imprimis* (Hillsdale College) 26 (1997): 5.

77. Royal Dutch Medical Association, "Policy Directive on Euthanasia," quoted in P. V. Admiraal, "Euthanasia in the Netherlands," *Free Inquiry* 17 (Winter 1996/97): 5.

78. T. E. Quill, "Doctor, I Want to Die. Will You Help Me?" *JAMA* 270 (18 August 1993): 870–73.

79. T. E. Quill, *A Midwife Through the Dying Process*, p. 205.

80. T. E. Quill, "The Story of Diane," in M. P. Hamilton, *Terminal Illness and Assisted Suicide*, pp. 12–13.

81. C. W. Dugger, "Tug of Taboos: African Genital Rite vs. U.S. Law," *New York Times*, 28 December 1996, pp. 1, 9.

82. J. Gross, "Doctor at Center of Supreme Court Case on Assisted Suicide," *New York Times*, 2 January 1997, pp. B1, B4.

83. D. Callahan, quoted in ibid.

84. R. Doerflinger, "Slippery Slope in Action" (Letter to the Editor), *New York Times*, 7 January 1997, p. A16.

85. Quoted in ibid.

86. "Assisted Suicide and the Law" (Editorial), *New York Times*, 6 January 1997, p. A16.

87. R. A. Lindsay, "Assisted Suicide: Will the Supreme Court Respect the Autonomy Rights of Dying Patients?" *Free Inquiry* 17 (Winter 1996/97): 4–5.

88. L. Montgomery, "Medical Student Group Backs Assisted Suicide," *Free Press* (Detroit), 11 December 1996, pp. 1A, 7A; T. Howarth, "Study of Assisted Suicide High on Dioceses' Agendas," *Episcopal Life*, February 1997, p. 15.

89. Quoted in D. Bird, "A Christian Moral Perspective," in M. P. Hamilton, *Terminal Illness and Assisted Suicide*, p. 33.

90. Ibid., p. 31.

91. D. Westley, *When It's Right to Die*, pp. 168–69.

92. D. Humphry, "Why I Believe in Voluntary Euthanasia," Humphry Internet Essay. http://www.rights.org/~deathnet/Humphry_essay.html. HTML. Copyright, 1995, Derek Humphry; emphasis added.

93. F. Girsh, "Right to Die" (Letters), *U.S. News & World Report*, 3 October 1997, p. 6.

94. F. Girsh, quoted in W. J. Smith, "Death March," *National Review*, 23 February 1998, p. 34; emphasis added.

95. Quoted in P. Steinfels, "Doctor-Assisted Suicide," *New York Times*, 11 January 1997, p. 31.

96. R. Dworkin, "Assisted Suicide: The Philosophers' Brief," *New York Review of Books*, 27 March 1997, pp. 41, 43.

97. Ibid., p. 43; emphasis added.

98. Ibid., p. 42.

99. B. Eads, "A License to Kill," *Wall Street Journal Europe*, 10 September 1997, p. 6.

100. Ibid.

101. *Washington et al. v. Glucksberg*, 1997 WL. 348094; and *Vacco v. Quill*, 1997 WL. 348037.

102. R. Dworkin, "Assisted Suicide: What the Court Really Said," *New York Review of Books*, 25 September 1997, pp. 40–44.

103. Ibid., p. 44; emphasis added.

104. T. S. Szasz, *Insanity*, and *Cruel Compassion*.

105. "Court Rejects the Sale of Medical Marijuana," *New York Times*, 26 February 1998, p. A21.

106. L. Greenhouse, "Assisted Suicide Clears a Hurdle in Highest Court," *New York Times*, 15 October 1997, pp. A1, A16.

107. P. Steinfels, "Doctor-Assisted Suicide in Oregon: An Idea That Complicates Health Care for the Poor and Challenges Government Neutrality," *New York Times*, 7 March 1998, p. A7.

108. "Suicide Is Never Health Care" (Editorial), *Syracuse Herald-Journal*, 18 April 1997, p. A18; emphasis added.

109. "Oregon Doctors Caught Between State and Federal Rules on Assisted Suicide," *Syracuse Herald-Journal*, 19 November 1997, p. A11.

110. N. A. Lewis, "U.S. Won't Prosecute Doctors Who Aid Suicide Via Oregon Law," *New York Times*, 6 June 1998, p. A7.

111. Ibid.

112. "Overreaching on Assisted Suicide" (Editorial), *New York Times*, 17 September 1998, p. A30.

CHAPTER 6 PERVERTING SUICIDE

1. R. Proctor, *Racial Hygiene*, pp. 190, 193; and D. Pappas, "Recent Historical Perspectives Regarding Medical Euthanasia and Physician-Assisted Suicide," *British Medical Bulletin* 52 (1996): 390.

2. Dutch Criminal Code, Article 293, quoted in P. V. Admiraal, "Voluntary Euthanasia: The Dutch Way," in S.A.M McLean, ed., *Death, Dying, and the Law*, p. 114; also quoted in D. Pappas, "Recent Historical Perspectives Regarding Medical Euthanasia and Physician-Assisted Suicide," *British Medical Bulletin* 52 (1996): 390.

3. P. Singer, *Practical Ethics*, p. 216.

4. R. Michener, "Foreword," in A. V. Dicey, *Introduction to the Study of the Law of the Constitution*, p. xxii. See also *Valentine's Law Dictionary*, p. 372.

5. For example, see "County Seeks Medical Use of Seized Marijuana," *New York Times*, 28 November 1997, p. A28.

6. J. Branegan, "'I Want to Draw the Line Myself,'" *Time*, 17 March 1997, pp. 30–31.

7. P. V. Admiraal, "Euthanasia in the Netherlands," *Free Inquiry* 17 (Winter 1996/97): 7–8; emphasis added.

8. J. Branegan, "'I Want to Draw the Line Myself,'" *Time*, 17 March 1997, pp. 30–31.

9. J. H. Groenewoud et al., "Physician-Assisted Death in Psychiatric Practice in the Netherlands," *New England Journal of Medicine* 336 (19 June, 1997): 1795–1801; emphasis added.

10. Ibid.; emphasis added. See also L. Ganzini and M. A. Lee, "Psychiatry and Assisted Suicide in the United States," *New England Journal of Medicine* 336 (19 June 1997): 1824–26.

11. P. V. Admiraal, "Euthanasia in the Netherlands," *Free Inquiry* 17 (Winter 1996/97): 5.

12. Ibid., p. 6.

13. B. Keizer, *Dancing with Mister D.*, pp. 167, 251.

14. Ibid., p. 256.

15. Ibid.

16. Ibid., p. 258.

17. Ibid., p. 301.

18. J. Branegan, " 'I Want to Draw the Line Myself,' " *Time*, 17 March 1997, pp. 30–31.

19. H. Hendin, quoted in P. Conradi, "Dutch Are 'Bullied' into Euthanasia," *Times* (London), 16 March 1997, pp. 1–12.

20. W. L. Toffler and M. J. Edwards, "Physician-Assisted Suicide" (Letters), *New England Journal of Medicine* 335 (15 August 1996): 519.

21. B. Keizer, *Dancing with Mister D.*, p. 301.

22. E. Goodman, "Dutch Have Grappled with Assisted Suicides," *Syracuse Post-Standard*, 18 April 1997, p. A14.

23. Ibid.

24. P. V. Admiraal, "Voluntary Euthanasia: The Dutch Way," in S.A.M. McLean, ed., *Death, Dying, and the Law*, p. 114.

25. Ibid.; emphasis added.

26. Ibid.

27. N. Hentoff, "Death in the Netherlands," *National Right to Life News* 24 (24 March 1997): 13.

28. Ibid.

29. Quoted in ibid.

30. P. Singer, *Rethinking Life and Death*, p. 158.

31. Ibid., p. 146.

32. Ibid., p. 158.

33. A. Chase, *The Legacy of Malthus*.

34. See generally, S. H. Harris, *Factories of Death*.

35. R. Proctor, *Racial Hygiene*, p. 180.

36. M. S. Pernick, *The Black Stork*, pp. 14–15.

37. Ibid., p. 95; emphasis in the original.

38. Ibid.

39. Ibid., p. 194.

40. B. Muller-Hill, *Murderous Science*, p. 23; and T. M. Moore, "A Century of Psychology in Its Relationship to American Psychiatry," in J. K. Hall, ed., *One Hundred Years of American Psychiatry*, p. 467.

41. Quoted in R. Proctor, *Racial Hygiene*, p. 180.

42. F. Kennedy, "The Problem of Social Control of the Congenital Defective: Education, Sterilization, Euthanasia," *American Journal of Psychiatry* 99 (July 1942): 14, 16. See T. S. Szasz, *Cruel Compassion*, Chapter 4.

43. See generally, R. Proctor, *Racial Hygiene*. Many of my subsequent quotations are from this important source about medical policy in Nazi Germany.

44. Ibid., pp. 259, 260.

45. J. S. Peck, "Ernst Simmel, 1882–1947," in F. G. Alexander et al., eds., *Psychoanalytic Pioneers*, p. 380.

46. R. Proctor, *Racial Hygiene*, p. 268.

47. Ibid., pp. 270, 273.

48. Ibid., pp. 185–86.

49. Ibid., p. 188.

50. J. Silvers and T. Hagler, "In the Name of the Führer," *The Sunday Times Magazine* (London), 14 September 1997, pp. 32–42.

51. R. Proctor, *Racial Hygiene*, pp. 188, 207; emphasis added.

52. Ibid., p. 207.

53. B. Muller-Hill, *Murderous Science*, pp. 39–40; emphasis added.

54. W. Pfaff, "Eugenics, Anyone?" *New York Review of Books*, 23 October 1997, pp. 23–24; and J. Silvers and T. Hagler, "In the Name of the Führer," *The Sunday Times Magazine* (London), 14 September 1997, pp. 32–42.

55. R. Proctor, *Racial Hygiene*, p. 212.

56. A. Chase, *The Legacy of Malthus*.

57. R. Proctor, *Racial Hygiene*, p. 212.

58. T. S. Szasz, *Insanity*, and *Cruel Compassion*.

59. D. Pappas, "Recent Historical Perspectives Regarding Medical Euthanasia and Physician-Assisted Suicide," *British Medical Bulletin* 52 (1996): 390.

60. Ibid. The author cites the British Medical Association's report *Euthanasia* (1988) as her source.

61. R. Proctor, *Racial Hygiene*, pp. 190, 193; emphasis in the original.

62. J. A. Barondess, "Medicine Against Society: Lessons from the Third Reich," *JAMA* 276 (27 November 1996): 1657–61.

63. R. Proctor, *Racial Hygiene*, p. 18.

64. B. Muller-Hill, *Murderous Science*, quoted in Ibid., pp. 44, 55.

65. Ibid., p. 23.

66. R. Proctor, *Racial Hygiene*, pp. 190, 193; emphasis in the original.

67. R. Servatius, quoted in H. Arendt, *Eichmann in Jerusalem*, p. 64; emphasis added.

68. R. J. Lifton, *Nazi Doctors*, pp. 15–16.

69. T. S. Szasz, *The Therapeutic State*, and *Insanity*.

70. J. G. Bachman et al., "Attitudes of Michigan Physicians and the Public Toward Legalizing Physician-Assisted Suicide and Voluntary Euthanasia," *New England Journal of Medicine* 334 (1 February 1996): 303.

CHAPTER 7 RETHINKING SUICIDE

1. J. Ortega y Gasset, *Man and Crisis*, p. 79.

2. F. von Hayek, *The Constitution of Liberty*, p. 31.

3. H. C. Black, *Black's Law Dictionary*, p. 852.

4. *Union Pacific Railway Co. v. Botsford*, 141 U.S. 250, 251 (1891).

5. *Olmstead v. United States*, 277 U.S. 438 (1928), p. 479.

6. See T. S. Szasz, *Psychiatric Slavery*.

7. *Application of President and Directors of Georgetown College*, 331 F. 2nd, 1010 (D.C. Cir. 1964); emphasis in the original.

8. *Thor v. Superior Court (Andrews)*, 855 P.2d 375 (Cal. 1993); pp. 375, 376, 384. The court was citing *In re Osborne* (D.C. 1972) 294 A. 2d 372, 375, fn. 5.

9. E. Burke, "A Letter from Mr. Burke to a Member of the National Assembly in Answer to Some Objections to His Book on French Affairs" (1791), in E. Burke, *The Works of the Right Honorable Edmund Burke*, vol. 3, p. 315.

10. A. de Jasay, *Against Politics*, p. 219.

11. T. E. Quill and H. Brody, "Physician Recommendation and Patient Autonomy: Finding a Balance Between Physician Power and Patient Choice," *Annals of Internal Medicine* 125 (1 November 1996): 765.

12. Ibid., pp. 767–68; emphasis added.

13. H. C. Black, *Black's Law Dictionary*, p. 1217.

14. T. S. Szasz, *Ceremonial Chemistry*, p. 175.

15. Ibid.

16. W. J. Smith, *Forced Exit*, p. 6; emphasis added.

17. Ibid., pp. 247, 252; emphasis added.

18. S. M. Glick, "Unlimited Human Autonomy: A Cultural Bias?" *New England Journal of Medicine* 336 (27 March 1997): 954–56; emphasis added.

19. D. Callahan, quoted in P. Wilkes, "The Next Pro-Lifers," *The New York Times Magazine*, 21 July 1996, p. 22 *ff.*; emphasis added.

20. Ibid.; emphasis added.

21. W. Gaylin and B. Jennings, *The Perversion of Autonomy*, pp. 8, 126.

22. Ibid., p. 58.

23. Ibid., p. 30.

24. See T. S. Szasz, "The Moral Dilemma of Psychiatry: Autonomy or Heteronomy?" *American Journal of Psychiatry* 121 (December 1964): 521–28.

25. W. Gaylin and B. Jennings, *The Perversion of Autonomy*, p. 66.

26. Ibid., p. 10.

27. M. Henry, "The Heritage of Gerhart Niemeyer," *Intercollegiate Review* 33 (Fall 1997): 7.

28. W. Gaylin and B. Jennings, *The Perversion of Autonomy*, p. 10.

29. Cited in N. B. Cummings, "Termination of Dialysis," in V. E. Andreucci and L. G. Fine, eds., *International Yearbook of Nephrology*, p. 129.

30. C. H. Calland, "Iatrogenic Problems in End-Stage Renal Failure," *New England Journal of Medicine* 287 (17 August 1972): 334–35.

31. J. T. DiBianco, "The Hemodialysis Patient," in L. D. Hankoff and B. Einsidler, eds., *Suicide*, p. 293.

32. Ibid., pp. 293, 294.

33. See generally N. B. Cummings, "Ethical and Legal Considerations in End-Stage Renal Disease," in R. Schrier and C. W. Gottschalk, eds., *Diseases of the Kidney*, vol. 3, pp. 2839–73, and "Social, Ethical, and Legal Issues Involved in Chronic Maintenance Dialysis," in J. F. Maher, ed., *Replacement of Renal Function by Dialysis*, pp. 1141–58.

34. D. G. Oreopoulus, "Withdrawal from Dialysis: When Letting Die Is Better than Helping to Live," *The Lancet* 346: 3–4 (1 July 1965): 4; and N. B. Cummings, "Termination of Dialysis," in V. E. Andreucci and L. G. Fine, eds., *International Yearbook of Nephrology*, p. 123.

35. Ibid.; and L. Y. Agodoa and P. W. Eggers, "Renal Replacement Therapy in the United States: Data from the United States Renal Data System," *American Journal of Kidney Diseases* 25 (January 1995): 119–33.

36. C. Catalano and C. Marino, "Death from Suicide and Discontinuation of Renal Replacement Therapy: 23-Years' Clinical Experience," *Nephron* 73 (1996): 737–38.

37. T. S. Szasz, *The Second Sin*, p. 76.

38. L. Y. Agodoa and P. W. Eggers, "Renal Replacement Therapy in the United States: Data from the United States Renal Data System," *American Journal of Kidney Diseases* 25 (January 1995): 119–33.

39. L. M. Cohen, "Suicide, Hastening Death, and Psychiatry," *Archives of Internal Medicine* 158 (12 October 1998): 1975.

40. See chapter 4.

41. I. Kerridge, M. Lowe, and K. Mitchell, "Competent Patients, Incompetent Decisions," *Annals of Internal Medicine* 123 (1 December 1995): 878–81.

42. N. B. Cummings, "Ethical and Legal Considerations in End-Stage Renal Disease," in R. Schrier and C. W. Gottschalk, eds., *Diseases of the Kidney*, vol. 3, pp. 2860–61.

43. E. L. Bliss, "Anorexia Nervosa," in A. M. Freedman, H. I. Kaplan, and B. J. Sadock, eds., *Comprehensive Textbook of Psychiatry—II*, p. 1657.

44. H. Bruch, *Eating Disorders*, p. 269.

45. "Michener's Kidney Dialysis," *USA Today*, 13 October 1997, p. 2D.

46. B. Hilton, "Did James Michener Commit Suicide or Just Die?" *Syracuse Herald-Journal*, 5 November 1997, p. B6; emphasis added.

47. For a stimulating account of a humanized "biography" of God, see J. Miles, *God*.

48. *Griswold v. Connecticut*, 381 U.S. 479 (1965).

APPENDIX

1. T. Jefferson, "The Memoir" (1821), in T. Jefferson, *Memoir*, vol. 1, p. 125.

2. T. Jefferson, "Letter to Dr. Samuel Brown," 14 July 1813, in A. Koch and W. Peden, eds., *The Life and Writings of Thomas Jefferson*, p. 629.

3. L. Stephen, *The Science of Ethics*, pp. 391–92.

4. H. L. Mencken, *The Philosophy of Friedrich Nietzsche*, pp. 226–28. I thank Leo Elliott for calling this item to my attention.

5. F. Nietzsche, quoted in K. Jaspers, *Nietzsche*, pp. 325, 324.

6. W. Richter, *The Mad Monarch*, pp. 250–51.

7. For further details, see T. S. Szasz, *Law, Liberty, and Psychiatry*, pp. 48–53.

8. H. A. Johnson, "Osler Recommends Chloroform at Sixty," *The Pharos* 59 (Winter 1996): 24–26.

9. W. Osler, "The Fixed Period," in W. Osler, *Aequanimitas*, pp. 375–93.

10. H. A. Johnson, "Osler Recommends Chloroform at Sixty," *The Pharos* 59 (Winter 1996): 24–26. Subsequent quotations are from this source unless otherwise indicated.

11. H. Cushing, *The Life of Sir William Osler*, vol. 1, p. 669.

12. W. Osler, "The Fixed Period," in W. Osler, *Aequanimitas*, p. 382.

13. Ibid.

14. A. Trollope, *The Fixed Period*. For a detailed discussion of the relation of this novel to the current scene, see K. Boyd, "Euthanasia: Back to the Future," in J. Keown, ed., *Euthanasia Examined*, pp. 72–82.

15. H. Cushing, *The Life of Sir William Osler*, vol. 2, p. 311.

Selected Bibliography

References to articles, reports, and other items appearing in journals, magazines, newspapers, and pamphlets are fully identified in the Notes. Books cited in the Notes only by author and title are identified more fully below.

Alexander, F. G., Eisenstein, S., and Grotjahn, M., eds. *Psychoanalytic Pioneers*. New York: Basic Books, 1966.

American Psychiatric Association. *Diagnostic and Statistical Manual of Mental Disorders—III*. 3rd ed. Washington, DC: American Psychiatric Association, 1980.

———. *Diagnostic and Statistical Manual of Mental Disorders—IV*. 4th ed. Washington, DC: American Psychiatric Association, 1994.

Amis, M. *Night Train*. New York: Harmony Books, 1997.

Andreucci, V. E., and Fine, L. G., eds. *International Yearbook of Nephrology, 1997*. New York: Oxford University Press, 1997.

Aquinas, T. *The Summa Theologica of St. Thomas Aquinas*. Literally translated by Fathers of the English Dominican Province. London: R. T. Washbourne, 1918.

Arendt, H. *Eichmann in Jerusalem: A Report on the Banality of Evil*. New York: Viking, 1963.

Arieti, S., ed. *American Handbook of Psychiatry*. 3 vols. New York: Basic Books, 1959–1966.

———. *American Handbook of Psychiatry*. 2nd ed. 6 vols. New York: Basic Books, 1974.

Aristotle. *The Basic Works of Aristotle*. Edited by Richard McKeon. New York: Random House, 1941.

Artaud, A. *Selected Writings*. Edited by Susan Sontag. Translated by Helen Weaver. New York: Farrar, Straus and Giroux, 1976.

Baechler, J. *Suicides*. 1975. Translated by Barry Cooper. New York: Basic Books, 1979.

Bartlett, J. *Familiar Quotations*. 12th ed. Edited by Christopher Morley. Boston: Little, Brown & Co., 1951.

Battin, M. P., and Lipman, A. G., eds. *Drug Use in Assisted Suicide and Euthanasia*. New York: Hawthorn Press/Binghamton, NY: Pharmaceutical Products Press, 1996.

Battin, M. P., and Maris, R. W., eds. *Suicide and Life-Threatening Behavior: Suicide and Ethics*. New York: Human Sciences Press, 1983.

Battin, M. P., and Mayo, D. J., eds. *Suicide: The Philosophical Issues*. New York: St. Martin's Press, 1980.

Beauchamp, T. L., and Walters, L., eds. *Contemporary Issues in Bioethics*. Encino, CA: Dickenson Publishing Co., 1978.

Becker, E. *The Denial of Death*. New York: Free Press, 1973.

Berger, R. *Government by Judiciary: The Transformation of the Fourteenth Amendment*. 1977. Indianapolis: Liberty Fund, 1997.

Berlin, I. *Four Essays on Liberty*. London: Oxford University Press, 1969.

Berrios, G. E., and Porter, R., eds. *A History of Clinical Psychiatry: The Origin and History of Psychiatric Disorders*. New York: New York University Press, 1995.

Black, H. C. *Black's Law Dictionary*. 4th ed. St. Paul, MN: West Publishing Company, 1968.

Blackstone, W. *Commentaries on the Laws of England: Of Public Wrongs*. 1752–1765. Boston: Beacon Press, 1962.

Bleuler, E. *Dementia Praecox or the Group of Schizophrenias* 1911. Translated by Joseph Zinkin. New York: International Universities Press, 1950.

Bonhoeffer, D. *Ethics*. Edited by Eberhard Bethge. New York: Macmillan, 1955.

Brody, B. A., ed. *Suicide and Euthanasia: Historical and Contemporary Themes*. Dordrecht, Neth.: Kluwer, 1989.

Bruch, H. *Eating Disorders: Obesity, Anorexia Nervosa, and the Person Within*. New York: Basic Books, 1973.

Brydall, J. *Non Compos Mentis: Or, the Law Relating to Natural Fools, Mad-Folks, and Lunatick Persons, Inquisited, and Explained, for Common Benefit*. London: I. Cleave, 1700. Facsimile reprint. New York: Garland, 1979.

Buchanan, A. E., and Brock, D. W. *Deciding for Others: The Ethics of Surrogate Decision Making*. Cambridge: Cambridge University Press, 1989.

Burdett, H. C. *Hospitals and Asylums of the World: Their Origin, History, Construction, Administration, Management, and Legislation*. 4 vols. London: J. & A. Churchill, 1891–1893.

Bureau of Justice Statistics Special Report. Washington, DC: U.S. Bureau of Justice, December 1987.

Burke, E. *The Works of the Right Honorable Edmund Burke*. 12 vols. Boston: Wells & Lilly, 1826.

Burleigh, M. *Death and Deliverance: Euthanasia in Germany, 1900–1945*. Cambridge: Cambridge University Press, 1994.

Burton, R. *The Anatomy of Melancholy*. 1621. London: Nonesuch Press, 1925.

Butterfield, H. *The Whig Interpretation of History.* 1931. New York: Norton, 1965.

Bynum, W. F., Porter, R., and Shepherd, M., eds. *The Anatomy of Madness: Essays in the History of Psychiatry.* 3 vols. London: Tavistock, 1985–1988.

Callahan, D. *The Troubled Dream of Life: Living with Mortality.* New York: Simon and Schuster, 1993.

Camus, A. *The Myth of Sisyphus, and Other Essays.* 1942. Translated by Justin O'Brien. New York: Vintage, 1955.

Carothers, J. C. *The African Mind in Health and Disease: A Study in Ethnopsychiatry.* Geneva: World Health Organization, 1953.

Cavan, R. S. *Suicide.* 1928. New York: Russell & Russell, 1965.

Chase, A. *The Legacy of Malthus: The Social Costs of the New Science of Racism.* New York: Knopf, 1977.

Cheyne, G. *The English Malady: Or, A Treatise of Nervous Diseases of All Kinds, as Spleen, Vapours, Lowness of Spirits, Hypochondriacal, and Hysterical Distempers, etc.* London: Strahan & Leake, 1733.

Clare, A. *Psychiatry in Dissent: Controversial Issues in Thought and Practice.* London: Tavistock, 1976.

Collinson, G. D. *A Treatise on the Law Concerning Idiots, Lunatics, and Other Persons Non Compotes Mentis.* London: W. Reed, 1812.

Colt, G. H. *The Enigma of Suicide.* New York: Summit Books, 1991.

Cornwell, J. *The Power to Harm: Mind, Medicine, and Murder on Trial.* New York: Viking, 1996.

Corwin, E. S. *The Constitution: And What It Means Today.* Princeton: Princeton University Press, 1954.

Cushing, H. *The Life of Sir William Osler.* 2 vols. London: Oxford University Press, 1925.

DeSimone, C. *Death on Demand: Physician-Assisted Suicide in the United States, A Legal Research Pathfinder.* Buffalo: William S. Hein, Co., 1996.

Dicey, A. V. *Introduction to the Study of the Law of the Constitution.* 1885/1915. Indianapolis: Liberty Fund, 1982.

Donne, J. *Biathanatos.* 1646. New York: Facsimile Text Society, 1930.

Douglas, J. D. *The Social Meanings of Suicide.* Princeton: Princeton University Press, 1967.

Downing, A. B., and Smoker, B., eds. *Voluntary Euthanasia.* London: Peter Owen, 1986.

Droge, A., and Tabor, J. D. *A Noble Death: Suicide & Martyrdom Among Christians and Jews in Antiquity.* New York: Harper/San Francisco, 1992.

Dublin, L. I. *Suicide: A Sociological and Statistical Study.* New York: Ronald Press, 1963.

Durkheim, E. *Suicide: A Study in Sociology.* 1897. Glencoe, IL: Free Press, 1951.

Dworkin, R. *Life's Dominion: An Argument About Abortion, Euthanasia, and Individual Freedom.* New York: Knopf, 1993.

Edwards, R. B., ed. *Ethics of Psychiatry: Insanity, Rational Autonomy, and Mental Health Care.* Amherst, NY: Prometheus Books, 1997.

Edwards, R. B., and Graber, G. C., eds. *Bio-Ethics.* San Diego: Harcourt Brace Jovanovich, 1988.

The Encyclopedia of Philosophy. Edited by Paul Edwards. 8 vols. New York: Macmillan/Collier, 1967.

Encyclopedia of the Social Sciences, International. Edited by D. L. Sils. New York: Macmillan and Free Press, 1968.

Endler, N. S., and Persad, E. *Electroconvulsive Therapy: The Myths and the Realities*. Toronto, Can.: Hans Huber Publishers, 1989.

Engelhardt, H. T., Jr. *The Foundations of Bioethics*. 2nd ed. New York: Oxford University Press, 1996.

Epstein, R. A. *Mortal Peril: Our Inalienable Right to Health Care?* New York: Addison-Wesley, 1997.

Esquirol, J.E.D. *Mental Maladies: A Treatise on Insanity*. 1838. Facsimile of the English Edition of 1845. New York: Hafner, 1965.

Fedden, H. R. *Suicide: A Social and Historical Study*. London: Peter Davies, 1938.

Firestone, R. W. *Suicide and the Inner Voice: Risk Assessment, Treatment, and Case Management*. Thousand Oaks, CA: Sage Publications, 1997.

Flew, A. *Atheistic Humanism*. Buffalo: Prometheus Books, 1993.

Frankl, V. E. *Man's Search for Meaning: An Introduction to Logotherapy*. 1959. 3rd ed. Translated by Ilse Lasch. New York: Simon and Schuster/Torchbook, 1984.

———. *The Doctor of the Soul: From Psychotherapy to Logotherapy*. 1955. 3rd ed. Translated by Richard and Clara Winston. New York: Vintage, 1985.

Freedman, A. M., Kaplan, H. I., and Sadock, B. J., eds. *Comprehensive Textbook of Psychiatry—II*. 2nd ed. Baltimore: Williams & Wilkins, 1975.

Freud, S. *The Standard Edition of the Complete Psychological Works of Sigmund Freud*. Translated by James Strachey. 24 vols. London: Hogarth Press, 1953–1974. Cited as SE.

Gaylin, W., and Jennings, B. *The Perversion of Autonomy: The Proper Uses of Coercion and Constraints in a Liberal Society*. New York: Free Press, 1996.

Gibbon, E. *The Decline and Fall of the Roman Empire*. 1787/1796. Abridged edition. Edited by Dero A. Saunders. New York: Penguin, 1981.

Glover, J. *Causing Death and Saving Lives*. Harmondsworth: Penguin, 1977.

Goethe, J. W. *Autobiography*. In *The Complete Works of Johann Wolfgang von Goethe*. Translated by John Oxenford. 10 vols. New York: P. F. Collier & Son, n.d.

———. *Dichtung und Wahrheit (Poetry and Truth)*. In *Gedenkausgabe der Werke, Briefe und Gespräche*. 24 vols. Zürich und Stuttgart: Artemis Verlag, 1962.

Goffman, E. *Asylums: Essays on the Social Situation of Mental Patients und Other Inmates*. Garden City, NY: Doubleday/Anchor, 1961.

Goldin, J., ed. *The Living Talmud: The Wisdom of the Fathers and Its Classical Commentaries*. New York: Mentor, 1957.

Gomez, C. F. *Regulating Death: Euthanasia and the Case of the Netherlands*. New York: Free Press, 1991.

Gorowitz, S., et al., eds. *Moral Problems in Medicine*. Englewood Cliffs, NJ: Prentice-Hall, 1976.

Guterman, N., ed. *The Anchor Book of Latin Quotations*. New York: Anchor Doubleday, 1990.

Halbwachs, M. *The Causes of Suicide*. 1930. Translated by Harold Goldblatt. London: Routledge, 1978.

Hall, J. K., ed. *One Hundred Years of American Psychiatry*. New York: Columbia University Press, 1944.

Hamilton, M. P., ed. *Terminal Illness and Assisted Suicide: Medical and Christian Moral Perspectives*. Cathedral Papers, No. 6. Washington, DC: Washington National Cathedral, 1993.

Hankoff, L. D., and Einsidler, B., eds. *Suicide: Theory and Clinical Aspects*. Littleton, MA: PSG Publishing Company, 1979.

Harris, R., and Paxman, J. *A Higher Form of Killing: The Secret Story of Chemical and Biological Warfare*. New York: Hill and Wang, 1982.

Harris, S. H. *Factories of Death: Japanese Biological Warfare, 1932–45, and the American Cover-Up*. London: Routledge, 1994.

Hatton, C. L., Valente, S., and Rink, A. *Suicide: Assessment and Intervention*. New York: Appleton-Century-Crofts, 1977.

Hayek, F. A. *The Constitution of Liberty*. Chicago: University of Chicago Press, 1960.

Heller, M. *Cogs in the Wheel: The Formation of Soviet Man*. New York: Knopf, 1988.

Hendin, H. *Suicide in America*. New and expanded edition. New York: Norton, 1995.

———. *Seduced by Death: Doctors, Patients, and the Dutch Cure*. New York: Norton, 1997.

Herbert, A. *The Right and Wrong of Compulsion by the State, and Other Essays by Auberon Herbert*. 1885. Edited and introduction by Eric Mack. Indianapolis: Liberty Press, 1978.

Higgs, R. *Crisis and Leviathan: Critical Episodes in the Growth of American Government*. New York: Oxford University Press, 1987.

Hinsie, L. E., and Campbell, R. J. *Psychiatric Dictionary*. 3rd ed. New York: Oxford University Press, 1960.

Hooff, A. J. van. *From Autothanasia to Suicide: Self-Killing in Classical Antiquity*. London: Routledge, 1990.

Hubbell, W. *Friends in High Places: Our Journey from Little Rock to Washington, D.C.* New York: William Morrow, 1998.

Hume, D. *Essays on Suicide and the Immortality of the Soul*. 1757. Introduction by John Vladimir Price. Bristol, UK: Thoemmes Press, 1992.

Humphry, D. *Final Exit: The Practicalities of Self-Deliverance and Assisted Suicide for the Dying*. New York: Dell, 1992.

Hunter, R., and Macalpine, I. *Three Hundred Years of Psychiatry, 1535–1860: A History Presented in Selected English Texts*. London: Oxford University Press, 1963.

Ingersoll, R. G. *The Works of Robert G. Ingersoll*. New Dresden Edition. Edited by Clinton P. Farrell. 12 vols. New York: C. P. Farrell, 1900.

Inoguchi, R., and Nakajima, T., with Pineau, R. *The Divine Wind: Japan's Kamikaze Force in World War II*. 1959. Westport, CT: Greenwood Publishers, 1978.

Jacobs, D., ed. *Suicide and Clinical Practice*. Washington, DC: American Psychiatric Association, 1992.

Jacobs, D., and Brown, H. N., eds. *Suicide: Understanding and Responding*. Madison, CT: International Universities Press, 1989.

Jasay, A. de. *Against Politics: On Government, Anarchy, and Order*. London: Routledge, 1997.

Jaspers, K. *Nietzsche: An Introduction to the Understanding of His Philosophical Activity*. 1936. Baltimore: Johns Hopkins University Press, 1997.

Jefferson, T. *Memoir, Correspondence, and Miscellanies, From the Papers of Thomas Jefferson*. Edited by Thomas Jefferson Randolph. 6 vols. New York: Gray & Bowen, 1830.

———. *Thomas Jefferson on Democracy*. Selected and arranged by Saul K. Padover. New York: Mentor, 1939.

Jung, C. G. *C. G. Jung Letters*. Edited by Gerhard Adler. Translated by R.F.C. Hull. 2 vols. London: Routledge & Kegan Paul, 1973–1976.

Keizer, B. *Dancing with Mister D*. Translated by Bert Keizer. London: Transworld Publishers, 1996.

Kennedy, R. *Race, Crime, and the Law*. New York: Pantheon, 1997.

Keown, J., ed. *Euthanasia Examined: Ethical, Clinical, and Legal Perspectives*. Cambridge: Cambridge University Press, 1995.

Kerr, A., and Snaith, P., eds. *Contemporary Issues in Schizophrenia*. London: Gaskell/Royal College of Psychiatrists, 1986.

Kevorkian, J. *Prescription: Medicide, The Goodness of Planned Death*. Buffalo, NY: Prometheus Books, 1991.

Kleinig, J. *Paternalism*. Totowa, NJ: Rowman and Allanheld, 1983.

Koch, A., and Peden, W., eds. *The Life and Selected Writings of Thomas Jefferson*. New York: Modern Library, 1944.

The Koran. Translated by N. J. Dawood. Baltimore: Penguin, 1968.

Kraepelin, E. *Lectures on Clinical Psychiatry*. 1904. New York: Hafner, 1968.

Krall, H. *Shielding the Flame: An Intimate Conversation with Dr. Marek Edelman, the Last Surviving Leader of the Warsaw Ghetto Uprising*. 1977. Translated by Joanna Stasinska and Lawrence Weschler. New York: Henry Holt, 1986.

Lecky, W.E.H. *History of European Morals, From Augustus to Charlemagne*. 1899. Vols. 1–2. New York: George Braziller, 1955.

Lewis, C. S. *God in the Dock: Essays on Theology and Ethics*. Edited by Walter Hooper. Grand Rapids, MI: William B. Eerdmans, 1970.

Lifton, R. J. *The Nazi Doctors: Medical Killing and the Psychology of Genocide*. New York: Basic Books, 1986.

Mackay, C. *Extraordinary Popular Delusions and the Madness of Crowds*. 1841/1852. New York: Noonday Press, 1962.

Macmurray, J. *Persons in Relation*. London: Faber and Faber, 1961.

McIntire, M. S., and Angle, C. R., eds. *Suicide Attempts in Children and Youth*. Hagerstown, MD: Harper & Row, 1980.

McLean, S.A.M., ed. *Death, Dying, and the Law*. Aldershot, UK: Dartmouth, 1996.

Magill, F. N., ed. *Masterpieces of World Literature in Digest Form*. New York: Harper & Brothers, 1949.

Maher, J. F., ed. *Replacement of Renal Function by Dialysis*. Dordrecht, Neth.: Kluwer Academic Publishers, 1989.

Masaryk, T. G. *Suicide and the Meaning of Civilization.* 1881. Translated by William B. B. Weist and Robert G. Batson. Chicago: University of Chicago Press, 1970.

Mason, J. K., and Smith, R.A.M. *Law and Medical Ethics.* 2nd ed. London: Butterworths, 1987.

Maudsley, H. *Responsibility in Mental Disease.* 4th ed. London: Kegan Paul, Trench & Co., 1885.

Mencken, H. L. *A Mencken Chrestomathy.* New York: Knopf, 1949.

———. *The Philosophy of Friedrich Nietzsche.* 1908. 3rd ed. Port Washington, NY: Kennikat Press, 1967.

Menninger, K. *Man Against Himself.* New York: Harcourt Brace, 1938.

———. *The Vital Balance: The Life Process in Mental Health and Illness.* New York: Viking, 1963.

———. *The Crime of Punishment.* New York: Viking, 1968.

———. *Whatever Became of Sin?* 1973. New York: Bantam, 1978.

Miles, J. *God: A Biography.* New York: Knopf, 1995.

Mill, J. S. *Autobiography of John Stuart Mill.* 1873/1924. New York: Columbia University Press, 1944.

———. *On Liberty.* 1859. Chicago: Regnery, 1955.

———. *The Collected Works of John Stuart Mill.* Edited by Ann P. Robson and John M. Robson. 24 vols. London: Routledge & Kegan Paul, 1963.

Miller, R. D. *Involuntary Civil Commitment of the Mentally Ill in the Post-Reform Era.* Springfield, IL: Charles C. Thomas, 1987.

Montaigne, M. de. *The Complete Essays of Montaigne.* 1580. Translated by Donald M. Frame. Stanford: Stanford University Press, 1957.

Montesquieu, B. de. *The Spirit of the Laws.* 1748. Translated by Thomas Nugent. 2 vols. New York: Hafner Press, 1949.

More, T. *Utopia and Other Writings.* New York: New American Library, 1984.

Muller-Hill, B. *Murderous Science: Elimination by Scientific Selection of Jews, Gypsies and Others, Germany 1933–1945.* New York: Oxford University Press, 1988.

Nathanson, B. N. *The Hand of God: A Journey from Death to Life by the Abortion Doctor Who Changed His Mind.* Washington, DC: Regnery, 1996.

Nietzsche, F. *Beyond Good and Evil.* 1886. Translated by Walter Kaufmann. New York: Vintage, 1966.

Noll, R. *The Aryan Christ: The Secret Life of Carl Jung.* New York: Random House, 1997.

Nuland, S. B. *How We Die: Reflections on Life's Final Chapter.* New York: A. A. Knopf, 1994.

Ogden, R. *Euthanasia and Assisted Suicide in Persons with Acquired Immunodeficiency Syndrome (AIDS) or Human Immunodeficiency Virus (HIV).* British Columbia, Can.: Perreault Goedman Publishing, 1994.

Ortega y Gasset, J. *Man and Crisis.* Translated by Mildred Adams. New York: Norton, 1962.

Orwell, G. *The Orwell Reader: Fiction, Essays, and Reportage.* Introduction by Richard R. Rovere. New York: Harcourt, Brace & World, 1956.

Osler, W. *Aequanimitas: With Other Addresses to Medical Students, Nurses and Practitioners of Medicine.* 3rd ed. Philadelphia: Blakiston, 1943.

The Oxford Dictionary of Quotations. 4th ed. Edited by Angela Partington. New York: Oxford University Press, 1992.

Parry-Jones, W. L. *The Trade in Lunacy: A Study of Private Madhouses in England in the Eighteenth and Nineteenth Centuries.* London: Routledge & Kegan Paul, 1976.

Perlin, S. *A Handbook for the Study of Suicide.* Oxford: Oxford University Press, 1975.

Pernick, M. S. *A Calculus of Suffering: Pain, Professionalism, and Anesthesia in Nineteenth-Century America.* New York: Columbia University Press, 1985.

———. *The Black Stork: Eugenics and the Death of "Defective" Babies in American Medicine and Motion Pictures Since 1915.* New York: Oxford University Press, 1996.

Pierson, J. L., and Conwell, Y., eds. *Suicide and Aging: International Perspectives.* New York: Springer, 1996.

Plato. *Laws.* Translated by A. A. Taylor. In *The Collected Dialogues of Plato, Including the Letters.* Edited by Edith Hamilton and Huntington Cairns. Princeton: Princeton University Press, 1973.

———. *Phaedo.* Translated by Hugh Tredennick. In *The Collected Dialogues of Plato, Including the Letters.* Edited by Edith Hamilton and Huntington Cairns. Princeton: Princeton University Press, 1973.

Portwood, D. *Common-Sense Suicide: The Final Right.* New York: Dodd, Mead & Company, 1978.

Posner, R. A. *Age and Old Age.* Chicago: University of Chicago Press, 1995.

Prado, C. G. *Rethinking How We Age: A New View of the Aging Mind.* Westport, CT: Greenwood Press, 1986.

———. *The Last Choice: Preemptive Suicide in Advanced Age.* Westport, CT: Greenwood Press, 1990.

Pritchard, C. *Suicide—The Ultimate Rejection? A Psycho-Social Study.* Buckingham, UK: Open University Press, 1995.

Proctor, R. *Racial Hygiene: Medicine under the Nazis.* Cambridge: Harvard University Press, 1988.

Quill, T. E. *Death and Dignity: Making Choices and Taking Charge.* New York: Norton, 1993.

———. *A Midwife Through the Dying Process.* Baltimore: Johns Hopkins University Press, 1996.

Reagan, L. J. *When Abortion Was a Crime: Women, Medicine, and Law in the United States, 1867–1973.* Berkeley: University of California Press, 1997.

Reznek, L. *The Philosophical Defence of Psychiatry.* London: Routledge, 1991.

———. *Evil or Ill?: Justifying the Insanity Defense.* London: Routledge, 1997.

Richter, W. *The Mad Monarch: The Life and Times of Ludwig II of Bavaria.* Translated by William S. Schlamm. Chicago: Regnery, 1954.

Robitscher, J. *The Powers of Psychiatry.* Boston: Houghton Mifflin, 1980.

Rosen, G. *A History of Public Health.* New York: MD Publications, 1958.

———. *Madness in Society: Chapters in the Historical Sociology of Mental Illness.* Chicago: University of Chicago Press, 1968.

Roy, A., ed. *Suicide*. Baltimore: Williams & Wilkins, 1986.

Ryn, C. G. *The New Jacobinism: Can Democracy Survive?* Washington, DC: National Humanities Institute, 1991.

St. John-Stevas, N. *Life, Death, and the Law: Law and Christian Morals in England and the United States*. Cleveland: World, 1961.

Sartorius, R., ed. *Paternalism*. Minneapolis: University of Minnesota Press, 1983.

Schrier, R. W., and Gottschalk, C. W., eds. *Diseases of the Kidney*. 6th ed. Boston: Little, Brown, 1996.

Scull, A., MacKenzie, C., and Hervey, N. *Masters of Bedlam: The Transformation of the Mad-Doctoring Trade*. Princeton: Princeton University Press, 1996.

Seneca. *The Stoic Philosophy of Seneca*. Translated by Moses Hadas. New York: Norton, 1958.

Seven Great Encyclicals. Glen Rock, NJ: Paulist Press, 1963.

Shavelson, L. *A Chosen Death*. New York: Simon and Schuster, 1995.

Shneidman, E. S. *The Suicidal Mind.* New York: Oxford University Press, 1996.

Singer, P. *Practical Ethics*. 2nd ed. Cambridge: Cambridge University Press, 1993.

————. *Rethinking Life and Death: The Collapse of Our Traditional Ethics*. New York: St. Martin's Press, 1994.

Slovenko, R. *Psychiatry and Criminal Culpability*. New York: Wiley, 1995.

Smith, R. *Trial by Medicine: Insanity and Responsibility in Victorian Trials*. Edinburgh: Edinburgh University Press, 1981.

Smith, W. J. *Forced Exit: The Slippery Slope from Assisted Suicide to Legalized Murder*. New York: Times Books/Random House, 1997.

Sprott, S. E. *The English Debate on Suicide: From Donne to Hume*. La Salle, IL: Open Court, 1961.

Steinbock, B., ed. *Killing and Letting Die*. Englewood Cliffs, NJ: Prentice-Hall, 1980.

Stengel, E. *Suicide and Attempted Suicide*. 1964. Revised edition. Harmondsworth: Penguin, 1983.

Stephen, J. F. *A History of the Criminal Law of England*. 1883. 3 vols. New York: Burt Franklin, n.d.

————. *Essays, by a Barrister*. London: Smith, Elder & Co., 1863.

————. *Liberty, Equality, Fraternity: Three Brief Essays*. Foreword by Richard A. Posner. Chicago: University of Chicago Press, 1991.

Stephen, L. *The Science of Ethics*. London: Smith Elder, 1882.

————. *The Life of Sir James Fitzjames Stephen*. 1985. South Hackensack, NJ: Rothman Reprints, 1972.

Stevenson, B., ed. *The Macmillan Book of Proverbs, Maxims, and Famous Phrases*. New York: Macmillan, 1948.

Storr, A. *Solitude: A Return to the Self*. New York: Free Press, 1988.

Strauss, M. B., ed. *Familiar Medical Quotations*. Boston: Little, Brown, 1968.

Sudak, H. S., Ford, A. B., and Rushforth, N. B., eds. *Suicide in the Young*. Boston: John Wright–PSG, 1984.

Szasz, T. S. *Ideology and Insanity: Essays on the Psychiatric Dehumanization of Man*. Garden City, NY: Doubleday Anchor, 1970.

————, ed. *The Age of Madness: A History of Involuntary Mental Hospitalization Presented in Selected Texts*. Garden City, NY: Doubleday Anchor, 1973.

———. *The Second Sin*. Garden City, NY: Doubleday Anchor, 1973.

———. *The Myth of Mental Illness: Foundations of a Theory of Personal Conduct*. 1961. Revised edition. New York: HarperCollins, 1974.

———. *Psychiatric Slavery: When Confinement and Coercion Masquerade as Cure*. New York: Free Press, 1977.

———. *The Therapeutic State: Psychiatry in the Mirror of Current Events*. Buffalo: Prometheus Books, 1984.

———. *Ceremonial Chemistry: The Ritual Persecution of Drugs, Addicts, and Pushers*. 1976. With a new preface. Holmes Beach, FL: Learning Publications, 1985.

———. *Insanity: The Idea and Its Consequences*. New York: Wiley, 1987.

———. *The Ethics of Psychoanalysis: The Theory and Method of Autonomous Psychotherapy*. 1965. With a new preface. Syracuse: Syracuse University Press, 1988.

———. *The Myth of Psychotherapy: Mental Healing as Religion, Rhetoric, and Repression*. 1978. With a new preface. Syracuse: Syracuse University Press, 1988.

———. *Psychiatric Justice*. 1965. With a new preface. Syracuse: Syracuse University Press, 1988.

———. *Schizophrenia: The Sacred Symbol of Psychiatry*. 1976. With a new preface. Syracuse: Syracuse University Press, 1988.

———. *The Theology of Medicine: The Political-Philosophical Foundations of Medical Ethics*. 1977. With a new preface. Syracuse: Syracuse University Press, 1988.

———. *Law, Liberty, and Psychiatry: An Inquiry into the Social Uses of Psychiatry*. 1963. With a new preface. Syracuse: Syracuse University Press, 1989.

———. *Sex by Prescription*. 1980. With a new preface. Syracuse: Syracuse University Press, 1990.

———. *The Untamed Tongue: A Dissenting Dictionary*. La Salle, IL: Open Court, 1990.

———. *Our Right to Drugs: The Case for a Free Market*. Westport, CT: Praeger, 1992.

———. *A Lexicon of Lunacy: Metaphoric Malady, Moral Responsibility, and Psychiatry*. New Brunswick, NJ: Transaction Publishers, 1993.

———. *Cruel Compassion: Psychiatric Control of Society's Unwanted*. New York: Wiley, 1994.

———. *The Meaning of Mind: Language, Morality, and Neuroscience*. Westport, CT: Praeger, 1996.

———. *The Manufacture of Madness: A Comparative Study of the Inquisition and the Mental Health Movement*. 1970. With a new preface. Syracuse: Syracuse University Press, 1997.

Tocqueville, A. de. *Democracy in America*. 1835–1840. Edited by Phillips Bradley. 2 vols. New York: Vintage, 1945.

Todorov, T. *Facing the Extreme: Moral Life in the Concentration Camp*. 1991. Translated by Arthur Denner and Abigail Pollak. New York: Henry Holt, 1996.

Tribe, L. H. *American Constitutional Law*. Mineola, NY: The Foundation Press, 1978.

Trollope, A. *The Fixed Period*. 1882. London: Penguin, 1993.

Tuke, S. *Description of the Retreat: An Institution Near York for Insane Persons of the Society of Friends, Containing an Account of Its Origin and Progress, the Modes of Treatment, and a Statement of Cases.* 1813. Introduction by Richard Hunter and Ida Macalpine. London: Process Press, 1964.

Valentine's Law Dictionary. Edited by William F. Anderson. San Francisco: Bancroft & Whitney, 1969.

Warren, J. C. *Etherization; With Surgical Remarks.* Boston: Ticknor, 1847.

Warren, O. L. *Negligence in New York Courts.* New York: Matthew Bender, 1978.

Webb, M. *The Good Death: The New American Search to Reshape the End of Life.* New York: Bantam Books, 1997.

Webster, C., ed. *Health, Medicine, and Mortality in the Sixteenth Century.* Cambridge: Cambridge University Press, 1979.

Webster's Third New International Dictionary (Unabridged). 1961.

Weir, R. F., ed. *Physician-Assisted Suicide.* Bloomington, IN: Indiana University Press, 1997.

Wells, H. G. *Love and Mrs. Lewisham.* 1899. New York: Charles Scribner's, 1924.

Werblowsky, R.J.Z., and Wigoder, G., eds. *The Encyclopedia of the Jewish Religion.* New York: Holt, Rinehart and Winston, 1965.

West, D. J., and Walk, A., eds. *Daniel McNaughton: His Trial and the Aftermath.* London: Gaskell, 1977.

Westcott, W. W. *Suicide: Its History, Literature, Jurisprudence, Causation, and Prevention.* London: H. K. Lewis, 1885.

Westley, R. *When It's Right to Die: Conflicting Voices, Difficult Choices.* Mystic, CT: Twenty-Third Publications, 1995.

Williams, M. *Cry of Pain: Understanding Suicide and Self-Harm.* London: Penguin, 1997.

Yochelson, L., ed. *Symposium on Suicide.* Washington, DC: George Washington University School of Medicine, 1967.

Zweig, S. *The Royal Game.* New York: Viking, 1944.

Author Index

Subject Index

About the Author

THOMAS SZASZ is Professor of Psychiatry Emeritus at the State University of New York Health Science Center in Syracuse. He is widely recognized as the world's foremost critic of psychiatric coercions and excuses and as a leading philosopher of liberty-and-responsibility. He is the author of twenty-four books, including *The Myth of Mental Illness* (1961), *Our Right to Drugs: The Case for a Free Market* (Praeger, 1992), and *The Meaning of Mind: Language, Morality, & Neuroscience* (Praeger, 1996).